Recent Advances in

Paediatrics
20

Recent Advances in Paediatrics 19
Edited by T.J. David

ISBN 0-443-064 31-8

ISSN 0-309-0140

2003

Recent Advances in

Paediatrics
20

Edited by

T. J. David MD PhD FRCP FRCPCH DCH

Professor of Child Health and Paediatrics,
University of Manchester;
Honorary Consultant Paediatrician,
Booth Hall Children's Hospital,
Royal Manchester Children's Hospital and St Mary's Hospital,
Manchester, UK

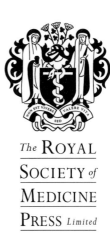

The ROYAL
SOCIETY *of*
MEDICINE
PRESS *Limited*

1 Wimpole Street, London W1G 0AE, UK
207 E Westminster Road, Lake Forest, IL 60045, USA
http://www.rsm.ac.uk

The authors are responsible for the scientific content and for the views expressed, which are not necessarily those of the Royal Society of Medicine, or of the Royal Society of Medicine Press Ltd. Medical knowledge is constantly changing. As new information becomes available, changes in treatment, procedures, equipment and the use of drugs become necessary. The editors and the publishers have, as far as possible, taken care to ensure that the information given in this text is accurate and up to date. However, readers are strongly advised to confirm that the information, especially with regard to drug usage, complies with current legislation and standards of practice.

British Library Cataloguing in Publication Data
A catalogue record for this book is available from the British Library

ISBN 1-85315-509-8

ISSN 0-309-0140

Commissioning editor - Peter Richardson
Editorial assistant - Gabrielle Lowis
Production by GM & BA Haddock, Midlothian, UK
Printed in Great Britain by Bell & Bain, Glasgow, UK

Contents

Preface

The aim of *Recent Advances in Paediatrics* is to provide a review of important topics and help doctors keep abreast of developments in the subject. The book is intended for the practising clinician, those in specialty training, and doctors preparing for specialty examinations. The book is sold very widely in Britain, Europe, North America and Asia, and the contents and authorship are selected with this very broad readership in mind. There are 13 chapters which cover a variety of general paediatric, neonatal and community paediatric areas. As usual, the selection of topics has veered towards those of general rather than special interest.

The final chapter, an annotated literature review, is a personal selection of key articles and useful reviews published in 2001. Comment about a paper is sometimes as important as the original article, so when a paper has been followed by interesting or important correspondence, or accompanied by a useful editorial, this is also referred to. As with the choice of subjects for the main chapters, the selection of articles has inclined towards those of general rather than special interest. There is, however, special emphasis on community paediatrics and medicine in the tropics, as these two important areas tend to be less well covered in general paediatric journals. Trying to reduce to an acceptable size the short-list of particularly interesting articles is an especially difficult task. Each topic in the literature review section is asterisked in the index, so selected publications on (for example) child abuse can be identified easily, as can any parts of the book that touch on the topic.

I am indebted to the authors for their hard work, prompt delivery of manuscripts and patience in dealing with my queries and requests. I would also like to thank my secretaries Angela Smithies and Val Smith, and Gill Haddock of the RSM Press for all their help. Working on a book such as this makes huge inroads into one's spare time, and my special thanks go to my wife and sons for all their support.

2002   ***Professor T.J. David***

University Department of Child Health, Booth Hall Children's Hospital,
Charlestown Road, Blackley, Manchester M9 7AA, UK
E-mail: t.david@netcomuk.co.uk

Heather Elphick Mark L. Everard

1

Noisy breathing in children

Recent studies using videos of children with wheeze and other forms of noisy breathing together with studies using acoustic analysis of breath sounds have challenged many assumptions about the use and validity of descriptions of noisy breathing such as 'wheeze'. It has long been known that 'all that wheezes is not asthma'. It is now clear all that 'wheezes' is not wheeze. While it is clear that accurate interpretation of audible sounds associated with breathing is a key component in the diagnostic and therapeutic process, it is also clear that the use of these terms is frequently imprecise. The loose usage of these terms by professionals, parents and children significantly diminishes their value in both the clinical and epidemiological arenas. The difficulties in obtaining agreement amongst clinicians when labelling different phenotypes of noisy breathing exhibited by patients has been highlighted in previous studies,[1,2] while a number of recent studies have clearly illustrated the difficulties parents have in accurately describing symptoms.

Since breathing is normally quiet, the onset of noisy breathing in childhood frequently engenders anxiety amongst parents and clinicians. Noisy breathing is extremely common in childhood and this is particularly true in early childhood. Prospective studies have suggested that as many as 48% of children wheeze during the first 6 years of life,[3-5] while other sounds such as stridor, snoring, snuffling and ruttling are all relatively common. An early 'baby check' study found that 30% of 298 infants under 6 months of age were reported as having noisy breathing in the previous week and 11% had noisy breathing from birth.[6] Abnormal noises may be present during the examination of a child

Dr Heather Elphick MB ChB MRCPCH MD
Research Fellow, Royal Melbourne Children's Hospital, Australia

Dr Mark L. Everard MB ChB VRCPCH DM (for correspondence)
Consultant in Paediatric Respiratory Medicine, Department of Respiratory Medicine, Sheffield
Children's Hospital, Western Bank, Sheffield S10 2TH, UK. Tel: +44 114 271 7400; Fax: +44 114 273 0522;
E-mail: meverard@sch.nhs.uk

as in the case of wheeze during an acute exacerbation of asthma or stridor during an episode of croup. However, in the out-patient setting, symptoms are frequently absent during the consultation and the clinician is dependent upon the history, usually provided by a carer, when attempting to assess the cause of the child's problems. Reliance on an accurate history is particular important in young children with respiratory symptoms in whom there are few objective tests available to clinicians.[7,8] Imprecise use of terms can result in under- or overinterpreting symptoms resulting in accurate diagnostic labelling and treatment. Similarly, epidemiological studies assessing the incidence and prevalence of symptoms such as wheeze are almost always reliant upon reports provided by the child's carer and figures such as 48% of children wheezing are probably significantly overestimating the incidence of true wheeze. Such studies have shaped our current understanding of the nature of wheezing illness in early childhood, but their validity is dependent upon the accuracy of symptom reporting.

The observation that the usage of descriptive terms for noisy breathing by clinicians is far from precise is not new, but recent studies have highlighted the importance of attempting to be precise with the use of terms such as wheeze. Studies using acoustic analysis techniques have started to clarify terminology and have identified sounds that are not covered by current medical jargon, while clinical studies using videos have highlighted the difficulties in describing phenotypes of noisy breathing and the extremely variable use of these terms by clinicians and the general public. In particular, it is clear that many parents use the term 'wheeze' to describe other respiratory noises, and indeed non-noise symptoms, during medical consultations. This is presumably because they feel that 'wheeze' is the 'correct' medical term for noisy breathing or that it is a term used to describe signs such as laboured breathing. The situation is worse for patients from non-English speaking backgrounds since the term 'wheeze' has no direct counter part in many languages.[9,10] Similarly, as noted above, it can be difficult to get clinicians to report sounds accurately and consistently. For example, many clinicians use the term 'wheeze' for the audible course, harsh low pitched noises (ruttles) frequently heard in young children because the vast majority of text books do not have a term for this sound leading to diagnostic and therapeutic errors. This lack of precision by clinicians means that even those few epidemiological studies in which 'doctor diagnosed wheeze' is used as a criterion are probably flawed.

The aim of this article is to describe some of the forms of noisy breathing in children and will include examples of the acoustic properties of these sounds, demonstrated using a computerized breath-sounds analysis technique. The implications of using accurate terminology for these noises, in terms of clinical practice and epidemiological research, will be discussed.

HISTORICAL CONSIDERATIONS

Sounds arising from the chest have historically been regarded as an important source of diagnostic information. The writings of the Hippocratic school in around 400 BC refer to 'splashing, creaking, wheezing and bubbling sounds' originating from the chest.[11] A clinical history and listening to the patient's breathing, if the patients exhibits noisy breathing during the consultation, were and still remain the most valuable aspects of the clinical assessment. Additional information could be obtained in some cases by placing an ear on the chest. Further information became available when the stethoscope was invented in 1816 by the French physician Laennec. To preserve the modesty of one of his female patients, he used a rolled-up narrow tube of paper rather than placing his ear on her chest and discovered that sounds from within the chest were amplified. Some 180 years later, interpretation of the sounds heard in this way remains very subjective. It is entirely dependent upon the clinicians hearing and their skill in interpreting the sounds they hear. Moreover, the stethoscope attenuates sounds above a frequency of approximately 1200 Hz limiting the range of sounds that may be heard.

The first attempts to interpret these sounds objectively took place in 1953 when McKusick carried out the first quantitative measurements of sounds emanating from the chest.[12] These experiments were the forerunner of today's computerised studies of acoustic analysis. While acoustic analysis of breath sounds has remained a relatively unglamorous and relatively peripheral aspect of respiratory research and clinical practice, technological advances over recent years are such that a number of manufacturers are designing and developing sophisticated 'electronic stethoscopes' that not only improve sound quality but that can also record and interpret these sounds. The most important development that has allowed this to happen has been the huge progress in computing power that now makes possible rapid analysis of the sounds recorded. Indeed, some devices now utilise 'real-time' presentation of data, a feature impossible only a few years ago. Some devices are able to record and interpret sounds over prolonged periods generating permanent records and graphical reports. It is likely that such devices will gradually enter routine clinical practice.

NOISY BREATHING AND RESPIRATORY SOUNDS – CURRENT TERMINOLOGY

Terms widely used for the abnormal audible noises generated during breathing include wheezing, stridor, snoring and a range of terms used for other noises generated in the upper airway such as stertor, snuffles, congestion, and rattling. Ruttles can now be added to this list (see below). All these sounds have characteristic features when subjected to computer analysis as do the sounds generated during a cough. In addition, there are adventitious sounds (sounds that are superimposed on normal breath sounds) such as crackles that cannot be heard unless using a stethoscope or microphone.

The terminology used to describe respiratory sounds has always been ambiguous and imprecise and indeed remains so in routine clinical practice. Nearly 200 years ago, Laennec,[13], in his 1819 *Treatise in the Diseases of the Chest* suggested the term *rale*, which, translated literally means 'death rattle'. The Latin equivalent of this term is *rhonchus*. He divided *rales* into 5 subcategories, each descriptive of the underlying pathology. These terms included: *rales humides*, or crepitations; *rales muqueux*, described as gurgling through sputum; *rales secs*, suggestive of 'the cooing of a wood pigeon'; and *rales sibilants*, or whistling or hissing. Robertson and Coope wrote a report 150 years later,[14] still trying to disentangle the confusion and ambiguity surrounding the terms used, particularly in the interpretation and translation from the original French terms used by Laennec. They recommended the use of the term 'adventitious' sounds, meaning those sounds that are not normally present and divided them into continuous sounds such as wheezes and discontinuous sounds such as crepitations.

More recently, a European Community funded project CORSA (Computerized Respiratory Sounds Analysis) working with a European Respiratory Society task force has attempted to standardize terminology further. This work has been summarized in a recent *European Respiratory Review*.[17] This working group again divided sounds recorded from the chest into continuous wheezes and discontinuous sounds which they called crackles which can be further sub-divided on the basis of characteristics such as pitch and duration. They did not recommend the use of the term rhonchi for low pitch 'wheezes' as had been suggested by an American Thoracic Society working party. Unfortunately, under this nomenclature the term wheeze is not limited to the musical expiratory musical sound audible to the naked ear that most clinicians would refer to as wheeze, but would include noises such as stridor because it is a 'continuous' sound.

COMPUTERISED ANALYSIS OF RESPIRATORY SOUNDS

As noted above, the use of digital, computerized analysis provides a technique that allows more rigorous analysis of noises generated within the chest than is possible with the ear alone. This approach has contributed significantly to our understanding of these sounds, and it is likely to start having an impact in the clinical arena. A database of the acoustic properties of sounds linked with audiovisual images would allow standardization of terminology, assist in training, and improve the precision of the usage of terms such as wheeze. It may also have a variety of clinical applications such as providing a useful non-invasive technique for the evaluation of infants and young children with pulmonary disease in whom conventional lung testing is difficult and confined to specialist centres. It has already been used as a means of assessing response to challenges, such as methacholine, with changes in breath sounds evident before the onset of wheeze.[15] Since it is now possible to observe these changes in real-time, this opens up the possibility that challenge testing could be simplified. Data can be recorded and analysed in a number of ways.[16,17]

A limited amount of commercial equipment is currently available. One sound recording, analysis and display process currently being used for research is the computer programme R.A.L.E. (Respiration Acoustics Laboratory Environment) system (Fig. 1) from PixSoft Inc., which was developed in collaboration with paediatrician Hans Pasterkamp.[18] A small sensitive contact sensor (EMT 25C, Siemens) is attached to the skin of the chest using a double-sided adhesive ring. Lung sounds can be recorded for up to 1 min, with the baby or child breathing normally. The signals are amplified and transmitted to an IBM-compatible personal computer via an analogue-to-digital converter. Other systems include the PulmoTrack system (Karmel Medical, Israel), the HELSA system (Pulmer Ltd Helsinki, Finland), and Sleep Sound (BEA, Belgium).

An example of the power of this technique has been to demonstrate clearly that the acoustic properties of wheeze and ruttles (see below) in young

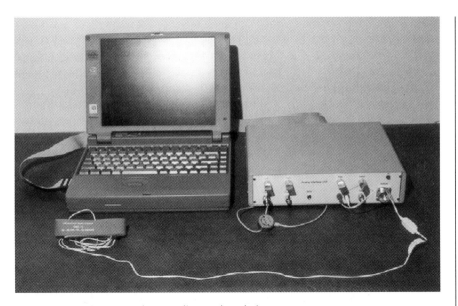

Fig. 1 R.A.L.E. lung sounds, recording and analysis.

children are quite distinct and they should be clearly differentiated if accurate diagnostic, therapeutic or epidemiological information is to be obtained.[19] The waveform display generated by this system represents the amplified output (V) from the contact sensor as a function of time (ms). Figure 2 represents a 100 ms segment of time during expiration. The waveform pattern for the wheezy baby has a very characteristic regular sinusoidal pattern, which contrasts with the non-sinusoidal, irregular and variable pattern noted in infants with ruttles. The Fourier power spectrum display (Fig. 3) is the plot of the log scale of the signal output, *i.e.* the signal intensity (dB) as a function of frequency (Hz) as calculated using a Fast Fourier Transformation technique. The upper line represents the breath sound recording; the lower line represents the background noise (cardiovascular and external). The normal power spectrum shows an exponential decay in intensity with increasing frequency. The power spectrum for the wheezy baby is characterized by distinct, sharp, narrow peaks of intensity at high frequencies with a width of about 10 Hz superimposed on the normal spectrum. As with the wheezing infants, there are abnormal peaks in the recordings from children with ruttles superimposed on the normal curve. However, in the case of ruttles, these peaks are multiple, diffusely distributed, and variable in size and shape. The most striking feature of this pattern is that it occurs in the lower frequency range < 600 Hz, where there is overall increased sound intensity compared to wheeze.

The clear differentiation of these two common sounds illustrates the potential power and objectivity of acoustic analysis.

WHEEZE

The term wheeze is used by clinicians on a daily basis and is probably the most commonly reported symptom of lower respiratory tract illness in infancy and early childhood. Therefore, it is surprising how few clinicians can accurately describe the sound. An audible wheeze is a continuous high pitched sound with a musical quality.[8,16] It is believed the term is derived from the old Norse word *hvaesa*, to hiss. It is important to recognise that there is no direct equivalent of the term wheeze in a number of languages.[9,10]

The musical nature of the sound is illustrated in Figure 3b with harmonics evident on the frequency/intensity plot. While predominantly an expiratory sound, a shorter inspiratory component is sometimes heard. Wheeze is a non-specific physical sign associated with restriction of airflow through narrowed airways. The mechanism of generation of the sound is thought to be due to narrowing of large central airways resulting turbulent flow causing oscillation

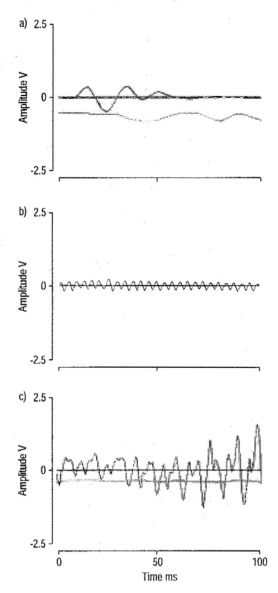

Fig. 2 Waveform patterns of: (a) normal child, (b) wheeze, and (c) ruttles.

of the airway walls,[18] although there is still some controversy regarding the exact mechanism. There are essentially two situations in which this occurs. Dynamic compression of the central airways associated with small airways disease. This results in wheezes of varying pitch occurring predominantly during expiration. Far less frequently, the wheeze maybe of fixed pitch occurring in inspiration and expiration suggesting a localised abnormality and narrowing of the trachea or main bronchus.

The use of the term wheeze remains central to both clinical practice and epidemiological research. Recurrent wheeze is frequently used to label children as having asthma and the symptom remains a corner stone of definitions of asthma. For instance, the international consensus statement on asthma defines it as recurrent wheeze and/or cough where asthma is likely

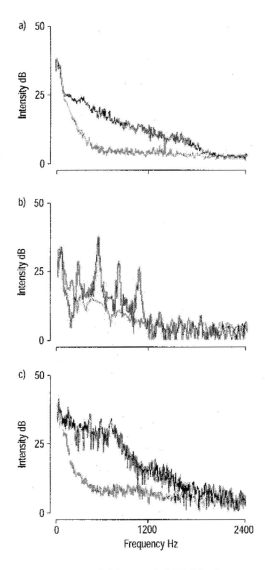

Fig. 3 Power spectrum patterns of: (a) normal child, (b) wheeze, and (c) ruttles.

and other rarer conditions have been excluded.[20] Our current understanding of wheezing illness has been shaped by large epidemiological studies undertaken in the 1980s and 1990s that have rediscovered that all that wheezes is not asthma and indeed the majority of children who wheeze in early childhood have what was known as wheezy bronchitis.[21] A number of recent studies have highlighted the fact that parents, professionals and children have difficulties in using the term in a consistent way. These studies and their implication for both clinical practice and research are discussed below.

RUTTLES

Many children with noisy breathing described as 'wheeze' instead make a coarse respiratory sound, which is lower in pitch than the wheeze, with a continuous coarse rattling quality and lacking any musical features.[8,21] The noise is termed 'ruttles' in Yorkshire and the north of England, although there are regional variations, including rattles, rustles and hustles. Characteristically, parents are able to feel this noise as a vibration over the baby's back in contrast to classical wheeze in which no such transmitted vibrations are evident. As noted above, objective breath sounds analysis has shown that this sound is quite distinct from wheeze.

Ruttles can be present from birth or commence after a bronchiolitic or other viral-induced respiratory illness. It is common in the first year of life, but rarely heard after 15–18 months of life. The underlying mechanism is unclear, but is likely to reflect excessive secretions in central and extra-thoracic airways or may be related to airways' tone. It often follows viral infections, which will induce glandular hyperplasia and disruption of cilial function.[22] This may lead to a relative excess of secretions in the airways and contribute to the presence of ruttles. The symptoms are frequently intermittent, can be exacerbated by viral infections, and do occur at night. Anecdotal reports suggest that, at their most extreme, infants have symptoms suggestive of obstructive sleep apnoea, though this is rare and resolves with time, as do the ruttles.

Since wheeze and ruttles are both common in early life, it is not surprising that occasionally they co-exist in the same child. However, it appears likely that they have different aetiologies and natural histories. It is also clear that they respond very differently to therapy which will influence both clinical practice and the outcome of clinical trials.[23] Computer analysis of the intensity of sound generated in young infants with wheeze and ruttles have confirmed the clinical impression that the sound of ruttles improves rapidly after the administration of ipratropium bromide while wheeze responds far less frequently. When there is a response, the magnitude of change in intensity of the wheeze is less than that seen with ruttles and the time course of action is much longer. The impact on ruttles may, in large part, explain why there is a widely-held belief that ipratropium is particularly useful in very young children with 'wheeze'. However, since ruttles generally resolve spontaneously in the second year of life, the short-term prognosis is good and re-assurance is generally all that is required.

STRIDOR

Stridor is less commonly confused with other forms of noisy breathing provided an accurate history is taken since is it is a continuous harsh sound occurring predominantly in inspiration. However, again, inaccurate assessment can result in such children being labelled as having recurrent wheeze and indeed being labelled as having asthma.

The term is taken from the Latin *stridulus* meaning creating, whistling or grating. Stridor is a sign of upper airway narrowing (larynx or extra-thorax) and, therefore, may be indicative of serious respiratory compromise. Stridor can be acute, usually of infectious origin, recurrent or chronic, often associated with congenital and acquired disorders of the larynx and vocal cords such as subglottic stenosis.

SNORING

Snoring is a common,[24,25] and frequently ignored, symptom in childhood. It results from partial obstruction of the upper airway, usually in the region of the oro-pharynx. The sound is typically irregular and inspiratory resulting from increased narrowing and vibration of the extra-thoracic airway during inspiration. Many children snore in their sleep without any significant disease or clinical problem. However, in approximately 0.5–3% of the population, the obstruction may be such that the child experiences obstructive sleep apnoea.[24,25] In its mildest form, this is manifest by brief obstructive apnoeas often terminating in loud inspiratory effort. More significantly, affected children will be aroused by the effects of the obstructive episode resulting in characteristic restless sleep. Typically, bedding is kicked off, children migrate around the bed and often they are sweaty. Frequent arousal results in poor quality, fragmented sleep leading to day-time tiredness and irritability. At its most marked, children will desaturate during apnoeas resulting in hypoxia and hypercarbia which can, if unrecognised, lead to pulmonary hypertension and cor pulmonale.

The most important cause of such problems in childhood is adenotonsillar hypertrophy[25] which may cause problems even in the first year of life. In children with relatively small upper airways, removal of tonsils and adenoids may relieve the symptoms even if they themselves do not appear excessively large. Other risk factors include relatively small airways, obesity, congenital malformations of the upper airways, and Down's syndrome.[25,26]

Assessment of a child with snoring includes a careful history and, where possible, observation of the apnoeic pauses. In children with a history suggestive of obstructive sleep apnoea, more detailed assessment should be undertaken. This can involve simple continuous pulse oximetry to the relatively expensive, but more informative, polysonography studies available in only a few paediatric centres in the UK. Children with episodic hypoxia will clearly benefit from intervention. It is also likely that a proportion of children with frequent arousals, but no episodes of documented hypoxia, will benefit from intervention, but there are no current guidelines as to which patients would benefit from intervention due to the lack of evidence. A recent study has indicated that snoring in early childhood, presumably associated with fragmented sleep, may have long-lasting effects on school performance.[27]

In has been shown that the sounds made by snoring adults with obstructive apnoeas are quantitatively different from those who snore alone and it has been suggested that overnight recordings may represent a significantly more cost-effective approach to the assessment of obstructive sleep apnoea than full polysonography.[28] It is likely to be sometime before the utility of this approach in children will be assessed.

Full discussion of obstructive sleep apnoea and its assessment is beyond the scope of this chapter.

OTHER ADVENTITIAL SOUNDS

Certain valuable respiratory noises (adventitial sounds) can be heard with the stethoscope, but not the naked ear. The most important of these are crackles which are discontinuous, 'crackling', adventitious sounds and can be divided into fine, or high pitched and coarse, or low pitched. They are intermittent and of short duration. The proposed mechanism for the generation of fine crackles is that they occur when a previously closed airway 'snaps' open when the appropriate combination of intrathoracic pressure, lung volume, tidal volume, and airflow occurs, resulting in a cascade of multiple superimposed brief noises in rapid succession. Fine crackles can be a non-specific feature of a range of pulmonary and cardiovascular causes including acute bronchiolitis, pulmonary oedema or interstitial lung disease. Coarse crackles are often related to airways' secretions, for example, in pneumonias or bronchiectasis. Several investigators, including Murphy, have identified features that will distinguish between fine and coarse crackles using acoustic analysis.[29]

PARENTAL REPORTING OF NOISY BREATHING

Few studies have explored the incidence and prevalence of 'noisy breathing' in great detail. Epidemiological studies have tended to focus on specific symptoms such as wheeze or associated sounds such as cough. There is some evidence that the responses to questions regarding wheeze are relatively repeatable compared with similar questionnaires related to cough, but even so there are considerable discrepancies in the responses to question regarding wheeze when re-administered to parents within 3 months.[30] Moreover, agreement between response to questions regarding wheeze and other respiratory symptoms when given by parents or their children are poor.[31] Such studies call in to question the recall of symptoms in both clinical practice and in questionnaire-based studies, but they do not provide any data regarding the accuracy of the use of terms such as wheeze. Further cause for concern was raised by the study of Cane et al. who found that 23% of parents attending a chest clinic did not consider noisy breathing to be a feature of wheeze and only 36% considered that wheeze referred specifically to noisy breathing. Difficulty in breathing and cough were felt to be important features that alerted them to the fact that their child was wheezing. The study also highlighted the low levels of agreement in the use of terms between the doctor in the clinic and the parent. In 39% of patients, parents used terms such as cough or difficulty breathing when wheeze was identified by the doctor.

Whistling was only mentioned by 11% of parents as a feature of wheeze, while only 1% reported that a whistling sound was present when their child wheezed. The authors highlighted the fact that almost all epidemiological studies utilize whistling in their description designed to help parents recognise a wheeze. Moreover, most questionnaires only provide a yes/no option which is likely to force parents into choosing the positive option if children have had any form of noisy breathing. The ISSAC study is one of the very few that has attempted to address the question more objectively by administering a questionnaire then reassessing responses after subjects were able to watch a video. Published data have consistently found the prevalence of wheeze to fall once subjects have been shown videos of children wheezing,[9] once again suggesting that the frequency of wheeze is over-reported.

As noted above, few studies have attempted to look at the prevalence of different types of noisy breathing. One study assessing the prevalence of a variety of symptoms in 298 infants less than 6 months of age found that noisy breathing was very common, with 30% of parents reporting noisy breathing in the previous 24 h and 11% of the infants were said to have had noisy breathing from birth.[6] Unusually, the investigators explored the nature of the noisy breathing in more detail and found that stridor accounted for 1% and wheeze for only 2% of the total prevalence of noisy breathing. The vast majority of infants, therefore, did not wheeze, but had 'snuffly' or 'upper airway noises'. Many of these probably exhibited ruttles.

A recent study investigated the terminology used by parents in both hospital and community settings to describe their children's breath sounds.[21] A questionnaire-based interview was carried out with the parents of 92 children under the age of 18 months. Parents were allowed, without any prompting, to give a detailed description of their child's noisy breathing. Following this, the parents were shown an imitation and/or a video recording of a wheeze, a ruttle, and a stridor and were asked to choose the sound that most resembled the noise made by their child.

Figure 4 shows the frequency of the terms most commonly used by the parents. The most common word offered by parents was wheeze (65%). The second most common words were ruttle and rattle (40%), which had a highly significant correlation with the description of bubbling or breathing through fluid. Other chosen words included rustles, squeaks, whistles, snuffles, and snorts. More imaginative phrases included descriptions such as 'tiger roaring', 'like a Labrador', 'like a pair of bellows that's not very efficient', 'like a dirty phone-call', 'smokes 40-a-day', and 'like a little pig'.

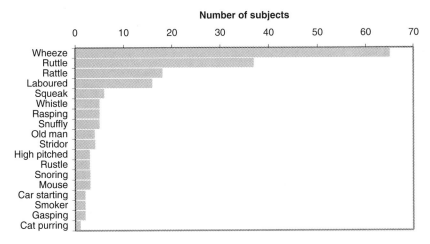

Fig. 4 Terms most commonly used by parents of infants to describe noisy breathing.[21]

When parents were asked what they meant by the word wheeze, the word 'whistle' was used to qualify the description of wheeze in only 8/65 (12%) cases. Four parents used the word 'tight' and three used 'high pitched'. On one occasion only, wheeze was described as a 'musical sound'. These findings were very similar to those of Cane et al.[16]

An interesting observation from this paper was that, without any prompting, parents were more likely to offer the word wheeze at the beginning of the interview. However, when shown video recordings, they were more likely to change their description to include ruttle. Of the parents questioned, 53% described their children as having wheeze during the initial interview; however, only 36% still used this term when shown video clips of children with wheeze and ruttles, representing a decrease of one-third of those originally using the term. The fall was greater still in the sub-group of parents recruited from the out-patient population. There was an increase in the use of the word ruttles from 40% during the interview to 81% after seeing the video clips. This reflects the degree of inaccuracy involved in the use of these terms in clinical practice, and may lead to over-diagnosis of wheeze in infants.

Cane and McKenzie further explored the parental interpretation of their children's respiratory symptoms using videos.[32] Five clinicians were able to agree on nomenclature for only 10 of 15 high quality selected video clips showing children with wheeze or other non-wheezing sounds such as stridor, snoring and stertor. A total of 190 parents of children aged less than 7 years were interviewed for the study and shown the 'gold standard' video clips. They formed three groups, those with a child diagnosed as having asthma or who had been observed to wheeze, those with other respiratory symptoms, and parents of children with no respiratory symptoms. Of the total, 27% described the non-wheezing sounds as wheeze or asthma while 8% described the examples of clear wheeze as other noises. Of parents of the 56 children with 'asthma' or who had been observed by doctors to wheeze, 20% did not recognize wheeze when shown the video clips. Interestingly, the authors suggest that parents were more likely to identify accurately the source of the respiratory noises than accurately describe the noise, particularly if English was not their first language. They also noted that in real life there may be significant overlap or co-existence of respiratory sounds in individual patients.

The authors concluded that an audiovisual presentation maybe helpful during consultations – a suggestion made by many others working in this field.[21,33] However, if the term wheeze is applied strictly to a very specific sound, audio files alone may be most appropriate since a parent watching a child asthma may identify the increased work of breathing they observe as wheeze rather than the associated audible noise.

IMPLICATION OF RECENT STUDIES

With no definitive gold standard for the definition of breath sounds in young children, terminology can be confusing for both medical staff and for parents. This highlights the need for accurate history taking. The responsibility lies with the doctor to ensure that interpretation of the language used by parents reflects accurately the noise that they mean to describe. Recent studies again highlight the need for high quality audiovisual material to help parents and clinicians. The use of video clips or audio files has been felt to be the most accurate method of assessing the children's respiratory noises and it has been suggested that this method may be useful in training health workers and in standardizing definitions of simple respiratory signs. If material is not available, it is often valuable to ask parents to video the child when they are symptomatic.

Subjective evaluation of breath sounds, however, is variable and intra-observer agreement on lung sound terminology has been found to fall somewhere between chance and total agreement, despite attempts to standardize nomenclature. The development of sophisticated analytical packages for the interpretation of breath sounds is likely to lead to more interest in this area of research in the future.

Clear and unambiguous descriptions of noisy breathing in children are clearly vital if clinical and epidemiological studies are to be valid. The failure of epidemiological studies to distinguish between distinct types of respiratory noise may lead to significant over-reporting of wheeze and an overestimation of the prevalence of wheeze in the community. This has potentially important implications for clinical trials, as well as for the diagnosis and therapy of respiratory disease in children.

Key points for clinical practice

- A wheeze is a musical sound generated in central airways by peripheral airways obstruction.

- All that wheezes is not asthma.

- All that wheezes is not wheeze.

- The term wheeze is used by parents and doctors to describe a variety of distinct audible sounds and non-respiratory signs such as increase work of breathing.

- Coarse, predominantly low-frequency respiratory noises known as ruttles are very common in infants and very young children.

- Ruttles and wheeze are both common and can co-exist.

- There is a more pronounced response to anticholinergics amongst children with ruttles than those with wheeze.

- Computerized breath-sounds' analysis is becoming increasingly sophisticated and its usefulness in both clinical practice and in clinical research is likely to increase.

- The lack of precision in the use of the term wheeze calls into question the validity of questionnaire-based epidemiological studies.

- Audiovisual material of children with a variety of respiratory symptoms may prove to be the most valuable method of allowing parents to identify accurately the types of symptoms their child is experiencing.

References

1. Pasterkamp H, Montgomery MD, Wiebicke W. Nomenclature used by health-care professionals to describe breath sounds in asthma. *Chest* 1987; **92**: 346–352.
2. Spiteri MA, Cook DG, Clarke SW. Reliability of eliciting physical signs in examination of the chest. *Lancet* 1988; **1**; 873–875.
3. Park ES, Golding J, Carswell F, Stewart-Brown S. Pre-school wheezing and prognosis at 10. *Arch Dis Child* 1986; **61**: 642–646.
4. Sporik R, Holgate ST, Cogswell JJ. Natural history of asthma in childhood – a birth cohort study. *Arch Dis Child* 1991; **66**: 1050–1053.
5. Martinez FD, Wright AL, Taussig LM. Asthma and wheezing in the first 6 years of life. *N Engl J Med* 1995; **332**: 133–138.
6. Thornton AJ, Morley CJ, Hewson PH, Cole TJ, Fowler MA, Tunnacliffe JM. Symptoms in 298 infants under 6 months old, seen at home. *Arch Dis Child* 1990; **65**; 280–285.
7. Pryor MP. Noisy breathing in children: history and presentation hold many clues to the cause. *Postgrad Med* 1997; **101**: 103–112.
8. Phelan PD, Landau LI, Olinski A. (eds) *Respiratory Illness in Childhood*, 2nd edn. Oxford: Blackwell Scientific, 1982; 104–131.
9. ISSAC Steering Committee. World-wide variation in the prevalence of asthma symptoms: the International Study of Asthma and allergies in Childhood (ISSAC). *Eur Respir J* 1998; **12**: 315–335.
10. Cane RS, Ranganathan SC, McKenzie SA. What do parents of wheezy children understand by 'wheeze'? *Arch Dis Child* 2000; **82**: 327–332.
11. McKusick V. *Cardiovascular Sound in Health and Disease*. Baltimore, MD: Williams & Wilkins, 1958.
12. McKusic VA, Jenkins JT, Webb GN. The acoustic basis of chest examination. *Am Rev Tuberc* 1953; **72**: 12–34.
13. Forbes J. *A Treatise of the Diseases of the Chest*. London: Underwood, 1821.
14. Robertson AJ, Coope R. Rales, Rhonchi and Laennec. *Lancet* 1957; **2**: 417–423.
15. Pasterkamp H, Consunji-Araneta R, Oh Y, Holbroe J. Chest surface mapping of sounds during methacholine challenge. *Pediatr Pulmonol* 1997; **23**: 21–30.
16. Gavriely N. *Breath Sounds Methodology*. Boca Raton, FL: CRC Press, 1995.
17. Computerized Respiratory Sounds Analysis (CORSA): recommended standards for terms and techniques. *Eur Respir Rev* 2000; **10**: Review 77.
18. Pasterkamp H, Carson C, Daien D, Oh Y. Digital respirosonography: new images of lung sounds. *Chest* 1989; **96**: 1405–1412.
19. Elphick HE, Ritson S, Rodgers H, Everard ML. When a 'wheeze' is not a wheeze: acoustic analysis of breath sounds in infants. *Eur Respir J* 2000; **16**: 593–597.
20. Warner JO, Naspitz CK, Third international pediatric consensus statement on the management of childhood asthma. *Pediatr Pulmonol* 1998; **25**: 1–17.
21. Elphick HE, Sherlock P, Foxall G *et al*. Survey of respiratory sounds in infants. *Arch Dis Child* 2001: **84**: 35–39.
22. Folkerts G, Verheyen AK, Geuens GM, Folkerts HF, Nijkamp FP. Virus-induced changes in airway responsiveness, morphology and histamine levels in guinea pigs. *Am Rev Respir Dis* 1993; **147**: 1569–1577.
23. Elphick HE, Ritson S, Everard ML. Differential response of wheezes and ruttles to anticholinergics. *Arch Dis Child* 2002; **86**: 280–281.
24. Ali NJ, Pitson D, Stradling JR. Natural history of snoring and related behaviour problems between the ages of 4 and 7 years. *Arch Dis Child* 1994; **71**: 74–76.
25. Rosen C. Diagnostic approaches to childhood obstructive sleep apnoea hypopnoea syndrome. *Sleep Breath* 2000; **4**: 177–182.
26. Tasker C, Crosby JH, Stradling JR. Evidence for persistence of upper airway narrowing during sleep, 12 years after adenotonsillectomy. *Arch Dis Child* 2002; **86**: 34–37.
27. Gozal D, Pope Jr DW. Snoring during early childhood and academic performance at ages thirteen to fourteen years. *Pediatrics* 2001; **107**: 1394–1399.

28. Perez-Padilla J, Slawinski E, Difrancesco L, Feige R, Remmers J, Whitelaw W. Characteristics of the snoring noises in patients with and without occlusive apnoea. *Am Rev Respir Dis* 1993; **147**: 635–644.
29. Murphy RL, Holford SK, Knowler WC. Visual lung-sound characterization by time-expanded waveform analysis. *N Engl J Med* 1977; **296**: 968–971.
30. Peat JK, Toelle BG, Bauman A, Woolcock AJ. Reliability of a respiratory history questionnaire and effect of mode of administration on classification of asthma in children. *Chest* 1992; **102**: 153–157.
31. Wong TW, Yu TS, Liu JL, Wong SL. Agreement on responses to respiratory illnesses questionnaire. *Arch Dis Child* 1998; **78**: 379–380.
32. Cane RS, McKenzie SA. Parents' interpretation of children's respiratory symptoms on video. *Arch Dis Child* 2001; **84**: 31–34.
33. English M, New L, Peshu N, Marsh K. Video assessment of simple respiratory signs. *BMJ* 1996; **313**: 1528.

Ellen R. Wald

2

Sinusitis in children: diagnosis and management

DEFINITION

The term 'sinusitis' refers to non-specific inflammation of the sinuses that can have a viral, allergic or bacterial origin. Unfortunately, most physicians and patients use the diagnosis of sinusitis to indicate bacterial infection of the sinuses. Sinusitis has been somewhat arbitrarily divided into three separate groups depending on the duration of symptoms. Acute sinusitis implies that there is a bacterial infection of the sinuses and is defined by nasal and sinus symptoms that have been present at least 10 days (in most cases) and less than 30 days. Subacute sinusitis is defined by nasal and sinus symptoms lasting longer than 4 weeks and less than 12 weeks. There is very little information comparing acute and subacute sinusitis, and this may ultimately prove to be an arbitrary distinction that does not reflect aetiology, diagnosis or treatment. Chronic sinusitis is defined by symptoms of at least 12 weeks' duration. The precise cause of chronic sinusitis is often unknown and, as a result, there is controversy regarding the treatment of this condition.[1]

EPIDEMIOLOGY

Symptoms in the upper respiratory tract are the most common complaint seen in the paediatric office.[2] One of the greatest challenges facing paediatricians is to distinguish between viral upper respiratory infections, allergic rhinitis and sinusitis. Distinguishing between these diagnoses is complicated by the fact that both allergic rhinitis and viral upper respiratory infections predispose patients to developing acute or chronic sinusitis. Young children experience

Professor Ellen R. Wald MD
Chief, Division of Allergy, Immunology & Infectious Diseases, Children's Hospital of Pittsburgh, 3705 Fifth Avenue, Pittsburgh, PA 15213, USA
Tel: +1 412 692 7489; Fax: +1 412 692 8499; E-mail: walder@chp.edu

6–8 viral upper respiratory infections per year of which 5–13% are estimated to be complicated by an episode of acute bacterial sinusitis.[3–5] Allergic rhinitis also is extremely common with a prevalence approaching 20% by adolescence. Patients with allergic rhinitis have an increased incidence of abnormal radiographic images of the paranasal sinuses. It is not known if patients with allergic rhinitis and abnormal sinus images have a bacterial explanation for their sinus inflammation. It is essential that paediatricians recognize that both allergic rhinitis and viral upper respiratory infections are probably at least 10 times more common than acute bacterial sinusitis.

PATHOGENESIS

The maxillary and ethmoid sinuses form during the third to fourth gestational month and, although very small, are present at birth. The maxillary sinuses are unique because the outflow tract sits high on the medial wall of the sinus cavity impairing the effects of gravity on drainage. The ethmoid sinus is comprised of multiple air cells each of which drains through a small, independent ostium into the middle meatus. The narrow calibre of these draining ostia predispose to obstruction. The frontal sinus develops from an anterior ethmoid cell and moves to a position above the orbital ridge by the fifth or sixth birthday. The sphenoid sinuses are immediately anterior to the pituitary fossa and just behind the posterior ethmoids. Isolated involvement of the sphenoid sinuses is rare; they are usually infected as part of a pansinusitis. The osteomeatal complex is the area between the middle and inferior turbinates which represents the confluence of the drainage areas of the frontal, ethmoid and maxillary sinuses (see Fig. 1A). Within the osteomeatal complex there are several sites in which two mucosal layers come into contact. The cilia move in opposite directions. Accordingly, there may be retention of secretions at this site and the potential for infection even without a physical obstruction of the ostia.

PHYSIOLOGY

Three key elements are important to the normal physiology of the paranasal sinuses: (i) the patency of the ostia; (ii) the function of the ciliary apparatus; and (iii) integral to the latter, the quality of secretions. Retention of secretions in the paranasal sinuses is usually due to one or more of the following: obstruction of the ostia, reduction in the number or impaired function of the cilia or overproduction or change in the viscosity of secretions.

The factors predisposing to ostial obstruction can be divided into those that cause mucosal swelling and those due to mechanical obstruction (Table 1). Although many conditions may lead to ostial closure, viral rhinosinusitis and allergic inflammation are by far the most frequent and most important. When complete obstruction of the sinus ostium occurs, there is a transient increase in intrasinal pressure followed by the development of a negative intrasinal pressure. When the ostium opens again, the negative pressure within the sinus cavity relative to atmospheric pressure may allow the introduction of bacteria into the usually sterile sinus cavity. Alternatively, sneezing, sniffing, and nose blowing with altered intranasal and intrasinal pressures may facilitate the entry of bacteria from the posterior nasal chamber into the sinuses.

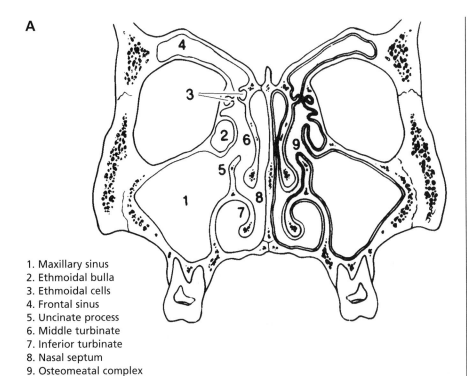

A

1. Maxillary sinus
2. Ethmoidal bulla
3. Ethmoidal cells
4. Frontal sinus
5. Uncinate process
6. Middle turbinate
7. Inferior turbinate
8. Nasal septum
9. Osteomeatal complex

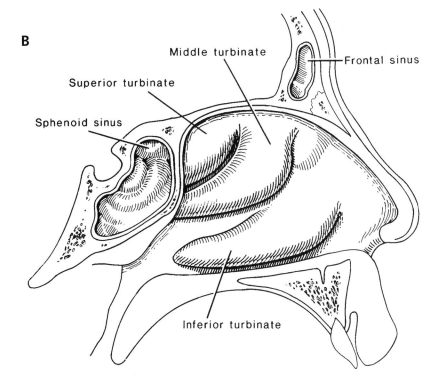

B

Middle turbinate

Frontal sinus

Superior turbinate

Sphenoid sinus

Inferior turbinate

Fig. 1 Coronal (A) and sagittal (B) sections of the nose and paranasal sinuses. The stippled area in (A) represents the osteomeatal complex.

Table 1 Factors predisposing to sinus ostial obstruction

Mucosal swelling		
	Systemic disorder	
		Viral URI
		Allergic inflammation
		Cystic fibrosis
		Immune disorders
		Immotile cilia
	Local insult	
		Facial trauma
		Swimming, diving
		Rhinitis medicamentosa
Mechanical obstruction		
		Choanal atresia
		Deviated septum
		Nasal polyps
		Foreign body
		Tumour
		Ethmoid bullae

The normal motility of the cilia and the adhesive properties of the mucous layer usually protect respiratory epithelium from bacterial invasion. The mucociliary apparatus may function abnormally because of either a direct cytotoxic effect on the cilia by respiratory viruses or a genetic defect in the microtubule structure of the cilia. The alteration of cilia number, morphology, and function may facilitate secondary bacterial invasion of the nose and the sinuses. Cilia can beat only in a fluid medium. Alterations in the mucus, as in cystic fibrosis or asthma, may impair ciliary activity. The presence of purulent material in the acutely infected sinus may also impair ciliary movement and further compound the effects of ostial closure.

SYMPTOMS AND SIGNS

Acute sinusitis has two common clinical presentations that distinguish it from an uncomplicated episode of viral rhinosinusitis (Table 2). The most common presentation involves persistent respiratory symptoms. In the context of acute bacterial sinusitis, persistent symptoms are those that last more than 10 days but less than 30 days and have not begun to improve. The 10-day mark separates simple viral rhinosinusitis from bacterial sinusitis and the 30-day mark separates acute sinusitis from subacute or chronic sinusitis. Most uncomplicated episodes of viral rhinosinusitis will last 5–7 days.[6,7] Although

Table 2 Clinical manifestations of acute sinusitis

Persistent symptoms	Nasal discharge or cough or both > 10 days and not improving
Severe symptoms	High fever (> 39°C) and purulent nasal discharge together for > 3–4 days

patients may not be asymptomatic by the tenth day, they are virtually always improved. Although upper respiratory symptoms in children are common, persistent symptoms lasting longer than 10 days are seen in a small minority (< 10%) of patients.[3] The symptoms should include either nasal discharge of any quality (thin or thick; clear, mucoid or purulent) and/or cough which must be present in the daytime (although it is often noted to be worse at night). Malodorous breath is often reported by parents of preschool children. Complaints of facial pain and headache are rare, although occasional painless morning eye swelling may have been noted by the parent. The child may not appear very ill and usually, if fever is present, it will be low grade. In this presentation, it is not the severity of the clinical symptoms but their persistence that calls for attention.

The second, less common presentation of acute sinusitis, is a 'cold' that seems more severe than usual. The severity is defined by a combination of high fever (at least 39.0°C) and purulent nasal discharge. The quality of nasal discharge undergoes frequent changes during the course of an uncomplicated viral upper respiratory infection. It begins as a watery discharge and becomes thicker, coloured and opaque after a few days. Most often, the nasal discharge will remain purulent for several days and then clear again to a mucoid or watery consistency before resolving. If fever is present at all during the course of an episode of viral rhinosinusitis, it is at the outset in association with other constitutional symptoms such as headache and myalgias.[6] Usually, the fever disappears and the respiratory symptoms begin. Accordingly, the combination of high fever and purulent nasal discharge for at least 3–4 days signals a secondary bacterial infection of the paranasal sinuses.[8] This group of patients may suffer from headaches behind or above the eye and occasionally experience peri-orbital swelling.

Patients with subacute or chronic sinusitis present with a history of protracted (more than 30 days and not improving) respiratory symptoms. Nasal congestion (obstruction) and cough (day and night) are most common. There is the frequent complaint of sore throat that results from mouth breathing secondary to nasal obstruction. Nasal discharge (of any quality) and headache are less common; fever is rare. It is important to distinguish between protracted symptoms and recurrent symptoms because of implications for both aetiology and treatment.

In general, the physical examination of children with either acute or chronic upper respiratory symptoms is most helpful in identifying conditions that may predispose to sinusitis; unfortunately, the examination cannot distinguish between viral upper respiratory infections and acute bacterial sinusitis.[9] Patients with nasal polyps, poor growth, clubbing of the fingers, barrel chest and respiratory findings may have cystic fibrosis. The immotile cilia syndrome is almost always associated with middle ear disease and 50% of patients have situs inversus. The presence of atopic dermatitis, intermittent wheezing, Morgan-Dennie lines (skin folds under the lower eyelid), or a nasal crease suggests an allergic diathesis. Patients with adenoidal hypertrophy can either predispose to sinusitis or masquerade as sinusitis. The adenoid cannot be assessed by routine examination, but rather requires either radiographic imaging or flexible endoscopy of the nasopharynx. Patients with immuno-deficiency may lack tonsillar tissue and other lymph nodes, have poor growth, clubbing of the fingers and other signs of infection.

DIAGNOSTIC METHODS

There is still significant controversy regarding the necessity for, and appropriate type of, radiographic imaging (plain film *versus* computerized tomography) for children with symptoms of sinusitis. Some recent national guidelines on the treatment of sinusitis have emphasized the role of the clinical diagnosis and moved away from the use of radiographic imaging in those patients with acute uncomplicated sinusitis.[2,10] However, the subcommittee on management of sinusitis of the American Academy of Pediatrics (AAP) has been conservative; they recommended that images are not necessary in children ≤ 6 years of age, but did not endorse the omission of radiographs in older children suspected to have sinusitis.[11] Plain films are appropriate in older children with recurrent acute sinusitis, vague symptoms, a poor response to antibiotic therapy, or a history of antibiotic hypersensitivity such that therapy poses additional risks. Radiographic findings in patients with acute bacterial sinusitis are diffuse opacification, mucosal thickening of at least 4 mm, or an air-fluid level. Using these radiographic criteria in the clinical setting of either 'persistent' or 'severe' acute sinusitis, sinus aspirates contained a high density of bacteria in 75% of children.[12,13]

It is noteworthy that computerized tomography (CT) scans are often significantly abnormal in children and adults with uncomplicated upper respiratory infections. CT scans in adult patients with an acute 'cold' virus showed significant abnormalities (including air-fluid levels) that resolved spontaneously.[14] In a study by Glasier *et al.*, almost 100% of young children who were undergoing CT examination for reasons other than sinus disease and who had an upper respiratory tract infection in the previous 2 weeks demonstrated soft tissue changes in their sinuses.[15]

The role for CT scans in patients with acute sinusitis is limited to those patients who present with signs of complicated disease. A CT scan should be considered in patients with proptosis, visual changes, limited extra-ocular movements, severe facial pain, notable facial swelling, deep-seated headaches, or a toxic appearance.[16] In children with chronic sinus symptoms, the CT scan remains the imaging technique of choice because of its high degree of anatomical detail. Most practitioners reserve imaging studies until after the completion of maximal medical therapy.

SINUS ASPIRATION

Although maxillary sinus aspiration is by no means a routine procedure, it can be safely performed by a skilled otolaryngologist using a transnasal approach. Current indications for maxillary sinus aspiration include: (i) failure to respond to multiple courses of antibiotics; (ii) severe facial pain; (iii) orbital or intracranial complications; and (iv) evaluation of an immuno-incompetent host. Material aspirated from the maxillary sinus should be sent for quantitative aerobic and anaerobic cultures (if possible) and Gram stain. The recovery of bacteria in a density of at least 10^4 colony forming units/ml is considered to represent true infection.[12] The finding of at least one organism per high power field on Gram stain of sinus secretions correlates with the recovery of bacteria in a density of 10^5 colony forming units/ml.

There has been some recent exploration into finding substitutes for sinus aspiration by less invasive methods including the performance of cultures of the middle meatus. Direct puncture of the maxillary sinuses, while remaining the gold standard for recovering bacteriological evidence, cannot be performed on younger children without sedation or general anaesthesia. Unfortunately, although middle meatal cultures do not involve direct puncture of the sinuses, they are still difficult to obtain in children who are awake. In studies on the microbiology of the middle meatus, samples were obtained in anaesthetized children who were undergoing otolaryngological procedures.[17] Furthermore, there may be a poor correlation between organisms recovered by culture of the middle meatus and those present in the sinuses, similar to the poor correlation between sinus aspirates and cultures of the throat and nasopharynx.[12] In a recent study,[17] it was shown that the most common organisms cultured from the middle meatus of a group of healthy children were the same as typical sinusitis pathogens. This casts serious doubt on the likelihood that obtaining cultures from the middle meatus will provide helpful information in individual cases.

MICROBIOLOGY OF SINUSITIS

Data on the microbiology of patients with acute (10–30 days) and subacute (30–120 days) illnesses have highlighted the important bacterial pathogens as *Streptococcus pneumoniae*, *Haemophilus influenzae* and *Moraxella catarrhalis*.[13,18] *S. pneumoniae* is most common in all age groups and accounts for 30–40% of isolates. *H. influenzae* and *M. catarrhalis* are similar in prevalence and account for approximately 20% of cases. Both *H. influenzae* and *M. catarrhalis* may be β-lactamase producing and, thereby, amoxicillin-resistant. Neither staphylococci nor respiratory anaerobes are commonly recovered from these patients.[12] Respiratory viral isolates include adenovirus, parainfluenza, influenza and rhinovirus in approximately 10% of patients. In children with chronic sinusitis, the role of bacterial agents is less clear. The results of cultures from children with chronic sinusitis have been extremely variable: a high percentage of patients have had either sterile cultures or known contaminants, and the presence of anaerobes has ranged from almost 0 to over 90%. The persistence of symptoms despite multiple courses of antimicrobials is counter to the notion that bacterial pathogens play a role in the aetiology of chronic sinusitis.[1]

MEDICAL TREATMENT

The clinical practice guideline developed by the AAP has recommended antibiotics for the management of acute bacterial sinusitis to achieve a more rapid clinical cure.[11] Evidence to support this recommendation was derived from a study comparing antimicrobial therapy to placebo in the treatment of children with both clinical and radiographic evidence of acute bacterial sinusitis.[19] Children between the ages of 2 and 16 years were stratified by age and clinical severity and randomized to receive amoxicillin, amoxicillin potassium clavulanate or placebo. On the third day of treatment, 45% of children treated with an antimicrobial were cured (complete resolution of respiratory symptoms) compared to 11% receiving placebo. On the 10th day of treatment, 79% of children receiving an antimicrobial were cured or improved compared with 60% of children receiving placebo. Approximately 50–60% of children will improve gradually without the use of antimicrobials; however, the recovery of an additional 20–30% is delayed substantially compared with children who receive appropriate antibiotics.

A recent study by Garbutt and co-workers has questioned the notion that children identified as having acute sinusitis on clinical grounds, without the performance of confirmatory radiographs, will benefit from antimicrobial therapy.[20] In this study, children with persistent respiratory symptoms, presumed to have sinusitis, were stratified by age and severity and randomized to receive either low-dose amoxicillin, low-dose amoxicillin/clavulanate or placebo. No differences were observed in outcome, either with regard to the timing of or frequency of recovery. The discrepancy in results between this investigation and the previous study may be attributable to several factors. The history of persistent respiratory symptoms (> 10 days and not improving) predicts abnormal sinus radiographs in nearly 90% of children less than 6 years of age.[19] However, this same history predicts the finding of abnormal sinus radiographs in only 70% of children aged 6 years and older. The Garbutt study included a large cohort of older children (mean age 8.0 years) who, therefore, may not have had sinusitis. While abnormal imaging studies cannot stand alone as diagnostic evidence of acute bacterial sinusitis without a strong clinical history, it is important to understand that a normal sinus radiograph is powerful evidence that bacterial sinusitis is not the cause of the clinical symptoms.[21] Without confirmatory radiographic evidence in children over the age of 6 years, as many as 30% of older children may have been misdiagnosed. Their inclusion in the study may obscure the anticipated differences in outcome of treated compared to untreated patients. In addition, Garbutt excluded the sickest patients (temperature > 39°C with facial pain and swelling), those most likely to benefit from antibiotics, potentially biasing the study in favour of no difference. Lastly, the choice of low-dose amoxicillin or amoxicillin/clavulanate, may be inadequate treatment for children who may harbour resistant organisms in their paranasal sinuses.

The clinical practice guideline published recently by the AAP concerning the diagnosis and management of sinusitis suggests that amoxicillin is a reasonable first choice for most cases of acute bacterial sinusitis in children.[11] This is especially true if the episode of acute bacterial sinusitis is uncomplicated, mild-to-moderate in degree of severity and if the patient has not recently (< 90 days) been treated with antimicrobial agents. While amoxicillin is preferred in most cases, there are several clinical situations in which a broader spectrum regimen is appropriate. These include: (i) failure to improve while being treated with amoxicillin; (ii) recent treatment with amoxicillin (< 90 days); (iii) attendance at day-care; (iv) the occurrence of frontal or sphenoidal sinusitis; and (v) presentation with very protracted (more than 30 days) symptoms. The antimicrobial with the most comprehensive coverage for these clinical situations is high-dose amoxicillin-potassium clavulanate (90/6.7 mg/kg/day in 2 divided doses). Alternative therapies for patients who are allergic to penicillin includes cefuroxime, cefpodoxime or cefdinir. In patients with serious hypersensitivity reactions to β-lactam antibiotics, azithromycin is a reasonable choice.

The emerging problem in the management of acute or recurrent sinusitis is infection caused by penicillin-resistant pneumococci. The frequency of penicillin-resistant pneumococci varies geographically and many isolates of pneumococci are resistant to other commonly used antimicrobials such as sulfamethoxazole-trimethoprim, loracarbef, cefixime, ceftibuten and to the macrolides. Therapeutic options include high-dose amoxicillin (80–90 mg/kg/day), high-dose amoxicillin/potassium clavulanate or clindamycin. Antibiotic selection should be guided by susceptibility results when available.

Patients with complications of sinusitis should be hospitalized and treated with parental antibiotic; subspecialty consultation may be appropriate. If penicillin-resistant pneumococci are suspected, cefotaxime (300 mg/kg/day in 4 doses), with or without vancomycin (40 mg/kg/day in 4 doses) should be given intravenously. Sinus aspiration should be performed to identify the infecting organism and aid in the selection of appropriate antimicrobial therapy.

Clinical improvement is prompt in nearly all children treated with an appropriate antimicrobial agent. Patients febrile at the initial encounter will become afebrile, and there is a remarkable reduction of nasal discharge and cough within 48 h.[8,19,22] If the patient does not improve, or worsens, in 48 h, clinical re-evaluation is appropriate. If the diagnosis is unchanged, an antimicrobial agent effective against β-lactamase-producing bacterial species and penicillin-resistant pneumococci should be prescribed. If the patient is still unresponsive, sinus aspiration should be considered in order to obtain precise bacteriological information.

The appropriate duration of antimicrobial therapy for patients with acute sinusitis has not been systematically investigated. All patients with uncomplicated acute sinusitis can be treated with 10–14 days of therapy. In those patients with chronic sinusitis, longer treatment courses have been used in an effort to avoid surgery. However, the use of antibiotic therapy for longer than a few weeks is not supported by any clinical studies, exposes patients to developing allergic hypersensitivity, and increases the risk of infection with resistant organisms.

Antibiotic prophylaxis as a strategy to prevent infection in patients who experience recurrent episodes of acute bacterial sinusitis has not been system-atically evaluated and is controversial.[22] A trial of antimicrobial prophylaxis may be appropriate if there is no treatable underlying disorder and there has been a history of responding to antibiotic therapy. Although antimicrobial prophylaxis has not been studied in patients with recurrent acute sinusitis, it has proved to be a useful strategy in reducing symptomatic episodes of acute otitis media in patients with recurrent ear disease.[23,24] Patients selected for a trial of antibiotic prophylaxis should have had at least three episodes of acute bacterial sinusitis in 6 months or four episodes in 12 months.[11]

Adjuvant therapies such as antihistamines, decongestants and anti-inflammatory agents have received little evaluation.[25] Antihistamines and decongestants have not been studied in patients with sinusitis, have as much potential to be harmful as they do to be helpful, and should not be used for this condition. The potential role of topical intranasal steroids as an adjunct to antibiotics in the treatment of acute bacterial sinusitis has recently been evaluated in children and adults.[26,27] The availability of intranasal steroids with a rapid onset of activity prompts consideration of these agents for the management of acute symptoms. To date, their beneficial effect has been extremely modest.[26] Nasal irrigation using either hypertonic or isotonic solutions has also been shown to have a positive effect in some patients. Saline nasal irrigation is inexpensive, readily available and devoid of side effects other than stinging discomfort from hypertonic solutions. Further prospective studies will be necessary to evaluate the role of adjuvant therapies in sinusitis.

COMPLICATIONS

Serious complications of acute sinusitis are uncommon and involve contiguous spread of infection to the orbit, bone or CNS (Table 3). Orbital complications are classified as inflammatory oedema (sympathetic effusion), subperiosteal abscess, orbital abscess, orbital cellulitis or cavernous sinus thrombosis. The first category of orbital involvement, referred to as inflammatory oedema, is not a true orbital complication. Peri-orbital soft tissue swelling occurs because the venous drainage of the tissues about the eye is impeded by a very congested ethmoid sinus. The veins that drain the face and lids pass next to or through the ethmoid sinus. When the ethmoid sinus is filled with pus and oedema, venous drainage is impaired. In this case, the infection is still confined to the sinuses. The lids may be very swollen and even erythematous but they are usually not tender. There is no proptosis and the extra-ocular movements are completely normal. This complication although not life threatening should be a signal to clinicians of a condition that may progress to a more serious form of orbital involvement. Accordingly, it should be followed closely and treated aggressively. The remaining orbital complications, subperiosteal abscess, orbital abscess, orbital cellulitis and cavernous sinus thrombosis are signalled by the presence of proptosis and impairment of the extra-ocular movements. Fortunately, these infections are rare these days.

Other complications of sinusitis are those that involve the bone and the CNS. Bony complications, such as Pott's puffy tumour, represent the formation

Table 3 Major complications of sinusitis

Orbital	
	Inflammatory oedema (preseptal or peri-orbital cellulitis)
	Subperiosteal abscess
	Orbital abscess
	Orbital cellulitis
	Optic neuritis
Osteomyelitis	
	Frontal (Pott's puffy tumour)
	Maxillary
Intracranial	
	Epidural abscess
	Subdural empyema or abscess
	Cavernous or sagittal sinus thrombosis
	Meningitis
	Brain abscess

of a subperiosteal abscess in the frontal bone adjacent to the frontal sinusitis. This is a result of an osteitis of the frontal bone. The CNS complications include brain abscess, subdural empyema, epidural empyema and meningitis. These complications are signalled by signs of increased intracranial pressure, meningeal irritation and focal neurological deficits in the case of intracranial infection.

It is worth noting that some complications of acute bacterial sinusitis are avoidable by the prompt and appropriate treatment of acute sinusitis. However, in a substantial number of children, the complication is the presenting illness without impressive or persistent preceding respiratory symptoms.

SURGICAL THERAPY

Patients with acute sinusitis hardly ever require surgical intervention unless they present with orbital or central nervous system complications. Rarely, sinus aspiration may be required both to ventilate and culture a sinus that has not responded to aggressive antimicrobial management. When patients with chronic sinusitis fail to improve with maximal medical therapy, sinus surgery might be considered. One academic otolaryngology centre has reported that complete evaluations for conditions that predispose children to chronic sinusitis combined with appropriate therapy directed toward these conditions reduced the number of surgical procedures to 3 over a 2-year period.[28] At present, the focus of surgical therapy is on the osteomeatal unit highlighted in Figure 1. Using an endoscope, most current surgical efforts attempt enlargement of the natural meatus of the maxillary outflow tract (by excising the uncinate process and the ethmoid bullae) and performance of an anterior ethmoidectomy. The outcomes of endoscopic sinus surgery are difficult to assess: all studies have been limited by retrospective designs and an absence of control groups. The precise population of children most likely to benefit from this surgery has not been delineated.

Key points for clinical practice

- Of viral upper respiratory infections, 5–13% are complicated by acute bacterial sinusitis in children.

- The most common presentation for acute sinusitis is with 'persistent respiratory symptoms' (nasal discharge or cough or both) that last more than 10 but less than 30 days and have not begun to improve.

- The other common presentation for acute sinusitis is with 'severe symptoms' of purulent nasal discharge and high fever (temperature > 39°C) for at least 3–4 consecutive days.

- The physical examination of children cannot distinguish between viral upper respiratory infections and acute bacterial sinusitis in most cases.

Key points for clinical practice (continued)

- There is still significant controversy regarding the necessity for, and appropriate type of, radiographic imaging (plain film *versus* computerized tomography) for children suspected to have sinusitis. Images are probably unnecessary for children ≤ 6 years of age with suspected acute bacterial sinusitis. Images may be necessary in older children.

- CT scans are appropriate in children with complicated sinus disease and those in whom surgical intervention is being considered.

- No image can stand alone as evidence of acute bacterial sinusitis. Abnormal images are produced by inflammation of the mucosa which may be caused by allergy, infection (viral or bacterial) or chemical or environmental irritation.

- Sinus aspiration (which reveals pus or bacteria in high density) is the best measure of acute bacterial sinusitis. Current indications for sinus aspiration include: (i) failure to respond to multiple courses of antibiotics; (ii) severe facial pain; (iii) orbital or intra-cranial complications; and (iv) evaluation of an immuno-incompetent host.

- The common causes of acute bacterial sinusitis include *Streptococcus pneumoniae, Haemophilus influenzae*, and *Moraxella catarrhalis.*

- Children with acute bacterial sinusitis that are treated with appropriate antibiotics recover more quickly and more often than children who are not treated.

- Amoxicillin is the drug of choice for acute uncomplicated bacterial sinusitis in children without risk factors for harbouring antibiotic resistant organisms (age < 2 years, attendance at day-care and recent receipt of antimicrobial agents). High-dose amoxicillin potassium clavulanate is appropriate when a child does not improve with amoxicillin or when there are risk factors that predispose to infection with resistant organisms.

- Neither prophylactic antimicrobials nor adjuvant therapies (antihistamines, decongestants and anti-inflammatory agents) can be recommended for children with acute bacterial sinusitis at this time due to inadequate and controversial data.

- The most common complications of acute sinusitis involve the orbit. 'Inflammatory oedema' or 'sympathetic effusion' is an example of peri-orbital swelling due to venous impedance secondary to a congested ethmoid sinus. More serious orbital complications (subperi-osteal abscess, orbital abscess, and orbital cellulitis) are signalled by proptosis, impairment of extra-ocular muscle movement or loss of visual acuity.

- Central nervous system complications of acute bacterial sinusitis are rare and include brain abscess, subdural and epidural empyema and meningitis.

References

1. Wald ER. Chronic sinusitis in children. *J Pediatr* 1995; **127**: 339–347.
2. Sinus and Allergy Health Partnership. Antimicrobial treatment guidelines for acute bacterial rhinosinusitis. *Otolaryngol Head Neck Surg* 2000; **123 (Suppl)**: S1–S32.
3. Aitken M, Taylor JA. Prevalence of clinical sinusitis in young children followed up by primary care pediatricians. *Arch Pediatr Adolesc Med* 1998; **152**: 244–248.
4. Ueda D, Yoto Y. The ten-day mark as a practical diagnostic approach for acute paranasal sinusitis in children. *Pediatr Infect Dis J* 1996; **15**: 576–579.
5. Wald ER, Guerra N, Byers C. Upper respiratory tract infections in young children: duration of and frequency of complications. *Pediatrics* 1991: **87**: 129–133.
6. Gwaltney Jr JM, Hendley JO, Simon G, Jordan Jr WS. Rhinovirus infection in an industrial population. II Characteristics of illness and antibody response. *JAMA* 1967; **202**: 494–500.
7. Gwaltney Jr JM, Buier RM, Rogers JL. The influence of signal variation, bias, noise, and effect size on statistical significance in treatment studies of the common cold. *Antiviral Res* 1996; **29**: 287–295.
8. Wald ER. Sinusitis. *Pediatr Ann* 1998; **27**: 811–816.
9. Lusk RP, Stankiewicz JA. Pediatric rhinosinusitis. *Otolaryngol Head Neck Surg* 1997; **117**: S53–S57.
10. McAllister WH, Porter BR, Kushner DC *et al*. Sinusitis in the pediatric population. In: *ACR Appropriateness Criteria*. Reston, VA: American College of Radiology; 2000. Available at <http//www.acr.org/departments/appropriateness_criteria/toc.html>. Accessed 23 February, 2001.
11. Subcommittee on Management of Sinusitis and Committee on Quality Improvement of the American Academy of Pediatrics. Clinical practice guideline: management of sinusitis. *Pediatrics* 2001; **108**: 798–808.
12. Wald ER, Milmoe GJ, Bowen A, Ledesma-Medina J, Salamon N, Bluestone CD. Acute maxillary sinusitis in children. *N Engl J Med* 1981; **304**: 749–754.
13. Wald ER, Reilly JS, Casselbrant M *et al*. Treatment of acute maxillary sinusitis in childhood: a comparative study of amoxicillin and cefaclor. *J Pediatr* 1984; **104**: 297–302.
14. Gwaltney Jr JM, Phillips CD, Miller RD, Riker DK. Computed tomographic study of the common cold. *N Engl J Med* 1994; **330**: 25–30.
15. Glasier CM, Mallory Jr GB, Steele RW. Significance of opacification of the maxillary and ethmoid sinuses in infants. *J Pediatr* 1989; **114**: 45–50.
16. McAlister WH, Kronemer K. Imaging of sinusitis in children. *Pediatr Infect Dis J* 1999; **18**: 1019–1020.
17. Gordts F, Abu Nasser I, Clement PA, Pierard D, Kaufman L. Bacteriology of the middle meatus in children. *Pediatr Otorhinolaryngol* 1999; **48**: 163–167.
18. Wald ER, Byers C. Guerra N. Subacute sinusitis in children. *J Pediatr* 1989; **XX**: 28–32.
19. Wald ER, Chiponis D, Ledesma-Medina J. Comparative effectiveness of amoxicillin and amoxicillin-clavulanate potassium in acute paranasal sinus infections in children: a double-blind placebo-controlled trial. *Pediatrics* 1986; **77**: 795–780.
20. Garbutt JM, Goldstein M. Gellman E, Whannon W, Littenberg B. A randomized, placebo-controlled trial of antimicrobial treatment for children with clinically diagnosed acute sinusitis. *Pediatrics* 2001; **107**: 619–625.
21. Kovatch AL, Wald ER, Ledesma-Medina J, Chiponis DM, Bedinyfield B. Maxillary sinus radiographs in children with nonrespiratory complaints. *Pediatrics* 1984; **73**: 306–308.
22. Gwaltney Jr JM. Acute community-acquired sinusitis. *Clin Infect Dis* 1996; **23**: 1209–1223.
23. Perrin JM, Charney E, MacWhinney Jr JB *et al*. Sulfisoxazole as chemoprophylaxis for recurrent otitis media: a double-blind crossover study in pediatric practice. *N Engl J Med* 1974; **291**: 664–667.
24. Casselbrant ML, Kaleida PH, Rockette HE *et al*. Efficacy of antimicrobial prophylaxis and of tympanostomy tube insertion for prevention of recurrent acute otitis media: results of a randomized clinical trial. *Pediatr Infect Dis J* 1992; **11**: 278–286.

25. Zeiger RS. Prospects for ancillary treatment of sinusitis in the 1990s. *J Allergy Clin Immunol* 1992; **90**: 478–495.
26. Barlan IB, Erkan E, Booker M, Berrak S, Basaran MM. Intranasal budesonide spray as an adjunct to oral antibiotic therapy for acute sinusitis in children. *Ann Allergy Asthma Immunol* 1997; **78**: 598–601.
27. Meltzer EO, Orgel HA, Backhaus JW *et al*. Intranasal flunisolide spray as an adjunct to oral antibiotic therapy for sinusitis. *J Allergy Clin Immunol* 1993; **92**: 812–823.
28. Parsons DS, Wald ER. Otitis media and sinusitis: similar diseases. *Otolaryngol Clin North Am* 1996; **29**: 11–25.

Colin Wallis

3

Recognition and treatment of atypical forms of cystic fibrosis

Cystic fibrosis (CF) is an autosomal recessive disorder and represents the commonest lethal inherited condition affecting white races. It is an ancient disease, but over the last 20 years there has been an acceleration in our understanding of the pathophysiology and the available treatment options.

For the majority of patients with CF, the diagnosis is clear. There is a classical phenotype of sinopulmonary disease and gastrointestinal manifestations with pancreatic insufficiency in 90%. The diagnosis is usually confirmed by a positive sweat test and two disease-causing mutations can be found in the CF gene if you look hard enough. In both the pancreatic sufficient and insufficient forms of 'classical' CF, changes to other organs often emerge with time – male infertility being one of the most consistent. As life expectancy has improved, so the list of associated complications has expanded. CF is now as much an adult disease as one of childhood, and it is the adult services that are learning more about CF complications such as osteoporosis, diabetes, liver failure, issues of pregnancy and even the CF menopause.

For many years, the sweat test has been the gold standard for the diagnosis of CF.[1] It has long been recognized, however, that there is a cohort of patients who clinically look like CF (or who have one or more typical features) but for whom the sweat test has not been reliably positive. For this group, it was always hoped that CF genotyping would provide diagnostic certainty. Two mutations within the gene for CF would mean cystic fibrosis; normal genes would exclude the diagnosis. But it has not worked out that simply. Indeed, in the decade since the discovery of the CF gene, the situation is probably even more confusing and the group of 'atypical' or 'unusual' cases is growing.[2]

Most clinicians who see children or adults with CF will have patients that fall into 4 groups: the first two are easy – those who have cystic fibrosis by anyone's

Dr Colin Wallis MD FRCPCH MRCP DCH
Consultant Paediatrician, Cystic Fibrosis Unit, Great Ormond Street Hospital for Children, Great Ormond Street, London WC1N 3JH, UK

Table 1 Why is a label of cystic fibrosis important?

- Explains a constellation of signs and symptoms
- Avoids unnecessary diagnostic testing
- Assists in planning appropriate treatment
- Guides prognostication and surveillance
- Informs antenatal decisions for future pregnancies
- Has implications for insurance and life-style

criteria, and clearly normal individuals. But there are two further groups – admittedly small but disproportionately challenging: (i) the individual who has two CF mutations (and maybe evidence of biochemical or electrical changes associated with the mutation), but does not develop the classical phenotype and may not have any symptoms or signs at all; and (ii) the patient who has one or a few features traditionally associated with CF, but in whom the sweat tests and genetic tests are either equivocal or negative.

It is important to diagnose someone with CF accurately (Table 1) and incorrect labelling must be avoided. As we enter the 21st century, CF is emerging as a disorder with a very wide phenotype – indeed not one disease but many. As the mysteries surrounding the convoluted route from genotype to phenotype are slowly unravelled, the handling of the atypical cases that are unearthed in the process needs clarification. This chapter looks at some of the factors that give rise to this challenging group of patients and discusses an approach to management.

WHY IS CYSTIC FIBROSIS SOMETIMES ATYPICAL?

THE COMPLEX ROUTE FROM GENETIC MUTATION TO CLINICAL DISEASE

The discovery of the gene for cystic fibrosis and the characterisation of its many mutations has led to the realisation that the disease we know as CF is far more complex than was anticipated. The road from two mutations to the final clinical phenotype is influenced by many factors along the way as depicted in Figure 1. A brief summary is provided below.

A THOUSAND CYSTIC FIBROSIS MUTATIONS

The cystic fibrosis transmembrane regulator gene (CFTR) codes for a protein of 1480 amino acids. The commonest mutation is the absence of a 3 base-pair sequence resulting in the loss of a phenylalanine residue at position 508 – designated ∆F508.[3] The remaining mutations are individually rare or unique, although some alleles tend to segregate within specific ethnic groups – for example, 36.2% of CF chromosomes in the Ashkenazi Jewish community carry the mutation W1282X, a gene with a frequency of < 1% in the UK.[4]

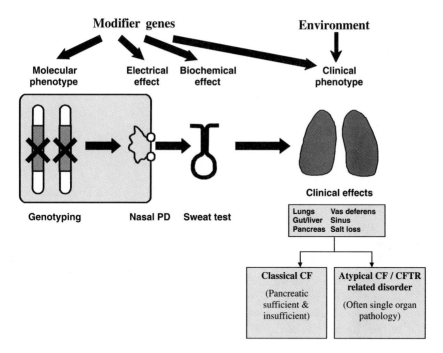

Fig. 1 A diagrammatic representation of the factors that can influence the path from two mutations (represented by the crosses) to a final phenotype that may be classical or atypical.

The wide distribution of mutations supports the ancient origins of this disease. Scientists from the early years following the discovery of the gene predicted that there may be as many as 10 different mutations. Little could they have anticipated that, by the end of that decade, nearly 1000 different mutations would be described and the list continues to grow. Every month further 'novel' mutations are reported.

CFTR mutations can be found throughout the length of the gene and have been classified into 5 different classes. This may produce a final product that is incomplete, complete but incorrectly packaged and processed (the most common defect), or a final protein product that is unstable or incapable of reaching the cell surface in sufficient numbers to be physiologically effective. This classification keeps things tidy for the scientists and may have bearing on future treatment developments.[5] Currently, however, it carries little clinical or diagnostic weight and will not be discussed further.

CFTR – A COMPLEX PROTEIN PRODUCT

The principal function of the CFTR appears to be as a cAMP-dependent chloride channel situated at the apical epithelial cell membrane. It is expressed in a wide range of tissues such as the airway, salivary and sweat glands, gastrointestinal tract, liver, pancreas and epidydimis.[4] Studies of the impact of a defective CFTR protein product have shown that the influence of this protein to maintain a stable salt and water milieu on the cell surface extends beyond regulation of chloride alone. Indeed, CFTR appears to have influence on amiloride-sensitive epithelial sodium channels, other chloride channels within the cell wall, and endocytosis and exocytosis in the CF pancreas.

Not only are the gene mutations proving a conundrum, but the final protein product behaves unpredictably and does not necessarily correlate with the final disease phenotype. It appears that when the genotype consists of two different mutations, some mutations are phenotypically dominant over others sometimes to positive effect for the final protein product.[6]

How does defective CFTR lead to pathology?

The path from defective CFTR to end-organ disease is still unknown. Several possibilities are currently being explored in an attempt to explain the lung disease:[7]

- CFTR may lead to a dehydrated airway surface liquid with: (i) the altered synthesis of surface proteins responsible for intrinsic mucosal defence such as defensins and lysosymes; (ii) an increase in the binding sites for *Pseudomonas aeruginosa* or a mucus that favours entrapment of bacteria such as Pseudomonads; (iii) a tendency to increased pro-inflammatory cytokines; or (iv) an alteration of mucins further impairing mucociliary clearance

- Defective CFTR may reduce the ability of the epithelial cells to ingest Pseudomonads

- Abnormal CFTR interferes with normal cell apoptosis and thus leads to a release of potentially toxic enzymes that play a role in disease pathogenesis

MODIFYING GENES

It is now recognised that modifying genes have significant influence on the behaviour of the CFTR gene, as well as the final protein product, the cell surface liquid and the final phenotype (Fig. 1). Modifying genes are likely to be numerous, unique to the individual, and represent an understudied area in the understanding of the pathophysiology of CF.[8] Consider them in two groups: (i) polymorphisms that fall within the CFTR gene; and (ii) genetic influences from elsewhere in the genome.

Modifying genes co-inherited within the CFTR gene

The mutation R117H is associated with CBAVD but does not cause lung disease – indeed it is commonly found in healthy males attending infertility clinics. If, however, the patient inherits a 5T variant in intron 8 (instead of the commoner 7T variant), then the likelihood of lung disease increases. This 5T variant reduces the splicing efficiency with lower levels of functioning CFTR and thus greater clinical impact.[9]

The A455E mutation is mostly associated with mild pancreatic disease. This mutation appears to have an interesting effect on the ΔF508 mutation if co-inherited, acting in a dominant fashion over ΔF508 and causing less severe lung disease.[6]

The clinical significance of polymorphisms such as the mis-sense mutation S1235R is also generating interest. This allele appears at a frequency that is significantly higher than that of many other CF mutations. When combined with a second CF mutation, the combination may cause disease. The question as to whether this mutation (and others like it) are rare polymorphism or a disease-forming mutation when combined with a known mutation leads to difficulties with genetic counselling, especially in prenatal cases.[10]

Modifying genes elsewhere in the genome

A gene that predisposes to meconium ileus

Meconium ileus is a presenting feature *in utero* or the early neonatal period in 10–15% of CF patients. There is a higher than expected rate of meconium ileus in siblings suggesting an inherited factor. Some investigators have postulated an association with the gene for haemochromatosis showing an increase in the carrier frequency of the haemochromatosis gene in children with meconium ileus and CF.[11]

More recently, the detection of a cystic fibrosis modifier locus for meconium ileus on human chromosome 19q13 has provided further evidence for a modifying gene that predisposes the carrier to this particular presentation of CF.[12]

Genetic variants of inflammation

Inflammation is a major player in the pathogenesis of lung disease in CF. There is a complex and highly individual soup of pro-inflammatory cytokines and protection factors that temper the final inflammatory response. Studies have looked at the impact of naturally occurring variants of a pro-inflammatory cytokine, tumour necrosis factor α (TNF-α), and the detoxifying enzyme glutathione S-transferase M1 (GSTM1).[13] A small study showed that the X-ray changes were significantly worse in those patients who were homozygous for the GSTM1 null allele and the absence of the TNF-α promotor polymorphism. We all have our own genetically determined and individual inflammatory system that could influence the pulmonary phenotype for those who also have CF.

Apparent absence of gene mutation

Finally, there are reports of patients with CF symptoms and a positive sweat test who do not appear to have any mutations in the CFTR gene even when the entire gene has been sequenced using denaturing gradient gel electrophoresis to screen all 27 exons and the intron–exon boundaries.[14] These finding suggest that CF may be caused by mutations within the promotor region of the CFTR gene, in one of the introns, or even in a distant controlling gene from an unrelated locus.[15]

OTHER MODIFYING PROTEINS

Researchers have recently focused on the role that other modifying proteins may have on the biochemical environment of the cell surface that could influence the CF phenotype and contribute to the spectrum of unusual forms. Some examples are given below.

Alternative chloride channels and protein kinases

The cell surface is known to have alternative chloride channels, the best studied of which carries the acronym ORDIC or ORCC (outward rectification of the current voltage relationship and increased open probability induced by depolarisation chloride channel).[7] In addition, there are a number of second-messenger pathways to cAMP (cGMP, calcium and protein kinase C). These alternative pathways are controlled to varying degrees by CFTR and provide a complicated orchestra of players contributing to the final electrophysiological environment on the cell surface of the CF epithelium.

Mannose-binding lectin

Mannose-binding lectin (MBL) is a key factor in innate immunity.[16] Investigators have shown interest in MBL variant alleles in cystic fibrosis addressing the possibility that they may predispose CF patients to recurrent infections and a worsening clinical course. Lung function appears to be significantly reduced in carriers of MBL variant alleles when compared with normal homozygotes, and there may be a correlation with the propensity to Pseudomonad infection. Presence of MBL variant alleles is, therefore, associated with poor prognosis and early death in patients with CF according to some authors.[17]

ENVIRONMENTAL FACTORS

Studies of siblings and twins (including identical twins) have confirmed that, although your genetic make-up is important in determining the course that your CF disease will follow, environmental factors account for the considerable differences in outcome between closely similar genotypes. Although there are many reports of phenotypic heterogeneity in twins (including monozygotic twins),[18] studies of large families demonstrate the striking variations present. In a highly consanguineous Bedouin tribe consisting of 29 subjects with CF, all homozygous for the mutation I1234V in exon 9, there was a wide variation of pulmonary disease, pancreatic insufficiency and electrolyte imbalance.[19]

Almost any external encounter, including psychological factors, can influence the clinical course. Examples are given below.

Infections

Pulmonary outcome in CF is influenced primarily by mucoid *P. aeruginosa* infection and only modestly by genotype. It is well known that the acquisition of Pseudomonads is associated with deterioration in lung function although the rate of progression of the lung disease is less predictable.[20] Viral lower respiratory tract infections in infancy can also produce a sustained negative impact and subsequent deterioration in lung function.[21]

Dietary influences

The associations between malnutrition, decreased vitamin and trace element absorption, and deteriorating lung function have been described.[22] The use of additional vitamin supplementation and enteric enzymes has a strongly positive impact on nutritional status.[23] Social circumstances are clearly central to effective dietary interventions.

Treatment and adherence to therapy

Treatment improves outcome. Failure to adhere to therapies could result in a deteriorating phenotype irrespective of the genetic background. Unfortunately, strict adherence does not guarantee good health which, understandably, is a cause of considerable distress for children and their families.

The timing of therapy is also important. Recent studies show that lung disease starts early, even before symptoms and signs are clinically evident.[24] A child growing up in a healthcare system where early intervention is available is likely to have an improved long-term outcome.

PHENOTYPE–GENOTYPE CORRELATIONS: THE PROMISE AND THE REALITY

The discovery of the CF gene led to the hope that phenotype–genotype correlation would be robust. By obtaining a genotype, one would be able to predict the type and perhaps even the course that your CF would take. It is disappointing to find that even though CF is a single gene disorder, there has been no convincing evidence that the risk of lung disease, liver disease, nasal polyposis or recurrent intestinal obstructive syndrome is related to any specific mutation.[25] There may be 'mild' mutations and 'severe' mutations and mild mutations may be dominant over severe ones, but the final effect on the phenotype is far more complex.[8] There are a few possible exceptions to the general disappointment:

1. Pancreatic sufficiency has been linked to certain mutations (such as R117H and A445E) although insufficiency may emerge with time.

2. Patients homozygous for the ΔF508 mutation generally (but not exclusively) have a more severe phenotype in all affected organs when compared to CF patients with one ΔF508 mutation or none.

3. Mutations carrying a milder pancreatic phenotype may be associated with less abnormal sweat tests and perhaps a similarly mild effect on nasal potential difference responses.

4. The male reproductive tract appears to have a high need for functioning CFTR, but splice mutations (such as 3840+10kbC>T) allow for the production of sufficient CFTR that fertility is possible (although not guaranteed) as illustrated in Figure 2.

THE DEFINITION OF CYSTIC FIBROSIS

Who has cystic fibrosis? As discussed, two disease-forming mutations in the CFTR gene make it highly likely that a CF phenotype will emerge – sometimes from birth, but occasionally evolving with the passage of time. This author's

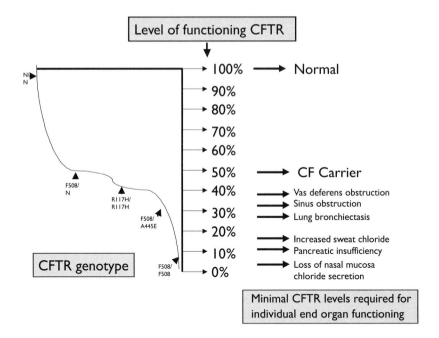

Fig. 2 This author's schematic representation of the possible relationship between genotype, levels of functioning CFTR and final clinical outcome.

example of a possible definition is outlined in Table 2. But just because you have two mutations in the gene does not necessarily mean that you will get the disease or that it will manifest in the classical way.

Any definition based on genetic criteria alone could lead to two obvious shortcomings: (i) one may label a patient who is clinically normal as having a disease just because of their genotype – an inaccurate assumption and one with considerable life-changing consequences; and (ii) the detection of a mutation from over a thousand possibilities is highly labour-intensive and only available in selected centres. Just because one cannot find the gene mutation in a patient who has symptoms of CF and would benefit from therapy is clearly wrong.

Most clinicians argue that the diagnosis of CF is a clinical decision – supported by biochemical and genetic tests.

Table 2 Cystic fibrosis is a disease that:

- Usually arises from two disease-forming mutations in the gene for CFTR on chromosome 7

- Results in changes to the fluid and electrolytes on cell surfaces

- Leads to an abnormal secretions and inflammatory response

- Predisposes to obstruction and infection

- Produces end-organ disease to tubular structures (upper and lower airways, vas deferens, gut, liver and pancreas)

MAKING THE DIAGNOSIS OF CYSTIC FIBROSIS

Since the 1950s, the sweat test has been the gold standard for confirming that a constellation of signs and symptoms was CF. Sweat chloride levels above 60 mmol/l are diagnostic (with only a few exceptions that are readily distinguished clinically from CF) and levels below 40 mmol/l are normal. This still holds true for the majority of patients, but the sweat test has moments of weakness. Notice that within the diagnostic and normal levels for sweat chloride lies an intermediate zone. Clinicians have always been aware of a small cohort of patients that have intermediate or fluctuating levels of sweat chloride and a suspect few in whom the sweat test is repeatedly normal.[1,2,26] The gold standard status afforded to the sweat test has slipped to silver class.

The advent of widely available genotyping of the CFTR gene held the promise that the fate of these atypical cases would be resolved. But this does not always happen and sometimes the situation is more confusing. Additional tests are required to either support or refute the diagnosis. Such tests could include measurements of nasal mucosal potential difference, detailed radiological examination of the chest or sinuses and pancreatic function testing.[27] But additional study often leads to a further increase in the number of atypical cases and the spectrum of disorders attributed to two mutations in the CFTR gene is expanding. CF is not one disease but many (Table 3).

THE EXPANDING CYSTIC FIBROSIS PHENOTYPE

There is a growing list of patients who have a phenotype that is not classically CF, but in whom more detailed biochemical and genetic studies provoke the question: 'could this be a form of unusual or mild or atypical CF?' Examples are listed in Table 4 and a selection are discussed briefly below.

Congenital bilateral absence of the vas deferens

Males with CF are almost all infertile with bilateral absence of the vas deferens. Infertility clinics are identifying a clinical syndrome of male infertility due to CBAVD in whom there is a high prevalence of CFTR mutations. Between 70–75% of males with CBAVD carry mutations in each CFTR gene – the commonest being ΔF508/R117H (without the 5T thymidine run in intron 8, see above).[28]

Table 3 Examples from the range of clinical features that can be associated with two mutations in the cystic fibrosis gene

- 'Classical CF' with pancreatic insufficiency
- Sinopulmonary disease, pancreatic sufficiency and positive sweat test
- Sinopulmonary disease and male fertility with normal sweat test
- Male infertility only
- Severe sinusitis and CBAVD
- Chronic pancreatitis only
- Allergic bronchopulmonary aspergillosis
- Positive sweat test only
- No clinical features including normal sweat chloride

Table 4 Examples of single organ disorders associated with an increased frequency of CFTR mutations

- Congenital bilateral absence of the vas deferens
- Chronic pancreatitis
- Chronic sinusitis
- Disseminated bronchiectasis
- Allergic bronchopulmonary aspergillosis
- Raised chymotrypsinogen in infancy

A proportion of these patients who are homozygous for CFTR mutations also have sweat chloride concentrations in the intermediate or abnormal range. Most have no other evidence of end-organ disease although, on careful questioning, a few reveal sinusitis or pulmonary symptoms.[29]

Disseminated bronchiectasis

Studies of disseminated bronchiectasis have determined a higher level of CFTR mutations than expected. Following a more detailed analysis of the CF gene, some have subsequently been determined to have two CF mutations and others have been found to carry the 5T variant.[30] It is likely that a number of these patients previously designated 'bronchiectasis of unknown origin' have insufficient levels of functioning CFTR to maintain lung health and are, in fact, examples of atypical CF.

Allergic bronchopulmonary aspergillosis (ABPA)

ABPA is found in patients with asthma and is also known to complicate the clinical course in patients with CF.[31] In a small study, the CF gene showed a higher level of mutation than could be expected in patients with ABPA suggesting again that CFTR may play a role in a less classical lung phenotype.[32]

Acute and chronic pancreatitis

Studies looking at adults presenting with either acute or chronic pancreatitis have revealed that a proportion have an unusual form of CF (almost always pancreatic sufficient),[26] but rarely demonstrate sinopulmonary disease or raised sweat chloride levels.[33]

IN SEARCH OF A NEW CLASSIFICATION FOR CYSTIC FIBROSIS

A US consortium has produced diagnostic criteria for CF which are summarised in Table 5.[34] These criteria hold true for many cases, but there are shortcomings as admitted by its members.[35] Perhaps two further categories of CF are required:

1. *A category for atypical cases.* The World Health Organization has recognised the need for a category that incorporates patients with atypical (often

Table 5 A US consensus panel approach to diagnostic criteria for cystic fibrosis

One or more clinical features consistent with CF
  Chronic sinopulmonary disease
  Gastrointestinal and nutritional abnormalities
  Salt loss syndromes
  Male urogenital abnormalities resulting in obstructive azoospermia

OR

A history of CF in a sibling

OR

A positive new-born screening test
AND an increased sweat chloride concentration by pilocarpine iontophoresis on two or more occasions
  or identification of two CF mutations
  or demonstration of abnormal nasal epithelial ion transport

single organ disease) who may or may not yield evidence for CFTR dysfunction (sweat test, nasal potential difference) or two CFTR mutations.[36] It is hoped that this additional category will appear in future editions of the *International Classification of Diseases*.

2. *A category for patients who have two CF mutations but have no evidence of clinical disease.* These patients may or may not have evidence for abnormal CFTR dysfunction. They may only show very subtle end-organ changes when subjected to detailed and sophisticated testing. For these individuals, it has been suggested that a well-established oncological concept is adopted.[37] Premalignant disease (*e.g.* carcinoma *in situ* of the cervix), which may never progress to cancer and which does not require immediate treatment, has long been recognised. In a similar light, two abnormalities in the CFTR region do not make the disease CF, although they may influence how we follow-up their owner. A classification that includes the concept of 'pre-CF' relieves the clinician from the falseness of 'all-or-nothing' decisions. No longer is there a need to decide whether someone is either normal or has a life-threatening disease of CF. There may be a slow evolution of CF-related complications in some individuals, whereas others may never proceed beyond the 'pre-CF' phase.

MANAGEMENT OF ATYPICAL CYSTIC FIBROSIS

The absence of a tight definition for CF and the failure of a reliable genotype–phenotype correlation are not necessarily a problem to the practicing clinician. Patients are individuals and require individualisation of their therapy. Treatment 'as if for CF' is an acceptable approach, ensuring that all is done to halt progression of pathology, but nothing is done that is superfluous and could impact negatively or impose unnecessary burden. Treat as indicated, monitor for anticipated problems, and intervene early to halt disease progression. Beware of the mild mutation – this is not necessarily an invitation for complacency in management and care.

When the genes are abnormal but the child is well

A 10-year-old girl had been tested *in utero* for CF as her older brother had been diagnosed with the disease. She was found to have two disease-associated mutations in each CFTR gene (N1303K and R117H associated with the 7T variant in intron 8). Sweat chloride levels have been repeatedly in the normal range. The patient is clinically asymptomatic and there is no evidence of lung, liver or pancreatic dysfunction

Management points

1. This patient could be considered as having 'pre-CF'. No therapy is required. A clinical phenotype could emerge in time, but she may never have disease. Genotype alone is an insufficient basis for the diagnosis of CF and a label as important as CF must be confined to someone with disease.

2. The need and frequency for long-term follow-up needs to be customised for the individual in conjunction with their paediatrician or physician.

3. Monitor for potential complications and intervene early to halt disease progression.

When the child looks like 'CF' but the tests do not confirm

A 15-year-old girl was diagnosed with CF at the age of two years following a history of chronic cough, asthma, foul smelling stools and failure to thrive. She is pancreatic insufficient and has sweat chloride levels that fluctuate between 50–70 mmol/l. Her height and weight are below the 5% and lung function tests reveal an FEV1 of 87%. She has grown *Staphylococcus* on cough swabs in the past and there is bronchial wall thickening on a CT scan of her chest. Extensive analysis of both CFTR genes in this patient (sequencing of all coding regions, flanking introns and the promoter, and Southern analysis for deletion/insertions) has failed to identify a mutation in either gene.

Management points

1. Ensure that other conditions that can masquerade as CF have been excluded. These would include some of the immunodeficiency states, ciliary abnormalities, rarer conditions such as Schwachman syndrome and certain allergic disorders that may present with diarrhoea, respiratory symptoms, and nasal polyps.

2. CF is a clinical diagnosis and if it looks like CF and responds to CF therapy, it should be treated aggressively as if CF. Geneticists are not yet in the position to say with certainty that because the mutations cannot be detected that the disease is excluded.

When the disease is atypical and so are the tests

A 15-year-old Caucasian girl had been attending the CF clinic since her diagnosis with CF at age 6 months. She had had a positive sweat test (chloride

65 mmol/l) performed during the work-up for a severe attack of bronchiolitis at 5 months of age. She had not required pancreatic enzyme replacement therapy and was thriving along the 50%. She had fallen out with her parents as she did not feel she had CF and was refusing all therapy. On examination, she was found to have a large nasal polyp. Further investigations were undertaken to try and firmly establish or refute the diagnosis. Repeat sweat testing showed an intermediate sweat chloride (45 mmol/l) with an equivocal result on testing her nasal potential difference (including chloride responses). A DNA analysis for 30 common CFTR mutations showed that she carried one ΔF508 mutation. Although she did experience intermittent episodes of wheezing, a CT scan did not show any evidence of lung pathology.

Management points

1. This patient probably fits the category of atypical CF – a form of CF increasingly diagnosed in older patients. Here, single organ features of CF (in this case nasal polyposis) are present, but there is incomplete corroborative test results to confirm a diagnosis of CF.

2. Treatment for atypical CF must be individualised. Deal with the complications, anticipate the early development of further complications, and introduce therapy as appropriate.

3. Do not impose therapeutic regimens and protocols that have been designed for the child with classical CF. They are inappropriate and burdensome.

4. A label of CF carries life-long consequences and must be reserved for those with the classical form. In time, it must be hoped that the atypical forms will acquire their due recognition as a separate entity

Key points for clinical practice

- Cystic fibrosis is a common, life-shortening autosomal recessive disorder. There is a classical phenotype consisting of purulent sinopulmonary disease and pancreatic malabsorption with infertility in males.

- A clinical suspicion of cystic fibrosis is usually confirmed by a positive sweat test and the detection of two disease-causing mutations in the cystic fibrosis transmembrane regulator (CFTR) gene.

- The discovery of many rarer mutations in the CFTR gene has revealed an ever-widening phenotype for this disease. Cystic fibrosis is now recognized to encompass a range of signs and symptoms (sometimes single organ) that previously would not have been considered within the cystic fibrosis umbrella.

- Many atypical forms of cystic fibrosis will have borderline or even normal sweat tests. Unusual gene mutations are not readily detected by routine CFTR analysis.

Key points for clinical practice (continued)

- It is anticipated that modifying genes will emerge as significant contributors to the range of clinical findings that occurs in cystic fibrosis – even in siblings who have the same genetic mutation.

- Atypical forms of cystic fibrosis can be usefully considered in two groups: (i) the individual who has two cystic fibrosis mutations (and maybe evidence of biochemical or electrical changes associated with the mutation), but does not develop the classical phenotype and may not have any symptoms or signs at all; and (ii) the patient who has one or a few features traditionally associated with cystic fibrosis, but in whom the sweat tests and genetic tests are either equivocal or negative.

- The management of atypical cystic fibrosis and the long-term follow-up should be customised for the individual, in conjunction with their paediatrician or physician.

- When there is evidence for two gene mutations in the CFTR gene but the child is well, no therapy may be required. However, this is not a mandate for complacency – a clinical phenotype may emerge with time. Monitor for potential complications and intervene early to halt disease progression.

- When the patient looks like cystic fibrosis but the tests do not confirm the diagnosis, ensure that other conditions that can masquerade as cystic fibrosis have been excluded.

- For patients where the disease is atypical and so are the tests, treatment must be individualised. Introduce treatment early to prevent complications but do not impose therapeutic regimens that are inappropriate and unnecessarily burdensome.

References

1. Littlewood JM. The sweat test. *Arch Dis Child* 1986; **61**: 1041–1043.
2. Massie J, Robinson P. Cystic fibrosis: the twilight zone. *Pediatr Pulmonol* 1999; **28**: 222–224.
3. Tsui LC. Molecular genetics of cystic fibrosis [Abstract]. *Isr J Med Sci* 1996; **32**: S1–S2.
4. Santis G. Basic molecular genetics. In: Hodson M, Geddes D. (eds) *Cystic Fibrosis*. London: Arnold, 2000; 27–48.
5. Zeitlin P. Novel pharmacologic therapies for cystic fibrosis. *J Clin Invest* 1999; **103**: 447–452.
6. Gan KH, Veeze HJ, van den Ouweland AM *et al*. A cystic fibrosis mutation associated with mild lung disease. *N Engl J Med* 1995; **333**: 95–99.
7. Alton E, Smith S. Applied cell biology. In: Hodson M, Geddes DM. (eds) *Cystic Fibrosis*. London: Arnold, 2000; 61–82.
8. Cutting G. Phenotype-genotype relationships. In: Hodson M, Geddes D. (eds) *Cystic fibrosis*. London: Arnold, 2000; 49–60.

9. Chu CS, Trapnell BC, Curristin S, Cutting GR, Crystal RG. Genetic basis of variable exon 9 skipping in cystic fibrosis transmembrane conductance regulator mRNA. *Nat Genet* 1993; **3**: 151–156.

10. Monaghan KG, Feldman GL, Barbarotto GM, Manji S, Desai TK, Snow K. Frequency and clinical significance of the S1235R mutation in the cystic fibrosis transmembrane conductance regulator gene: results from a collaborative study. *Am J Med Genet* 2000; **95**: 361–365.

11. Rohlfs EM, Shaheen NJ, Silverman LM. Is the hemochromatosis gene a modifier locus for cystic fibrosis? *Genet Test* 1998; **2**: 85–88.

12. Zielenski J, Corey M, Rozmahel R *et al*. Detection of a cystic fibrosis modifier locus for meconium ileus on human chromosome 19q13. *Nat Genet* 1999; **22**: 128–129.

13. Hull J, Thomson AH. Contribution of genetic factors other than CFTR to disease severity in cystic fibrosis. *Thorax* 1998; **53**: 1018–1021.

14. Mekus F, Ballmann M, Bronsveld I *et al*. Cystic-fibrosis-like disease unrelated to the cystic fibrosis transmembrane conductance regulator. *Hum Genet* 1998; **102**: 582–586.

15. Rozmahel R, Wilschanski M, Matin A *et al*. Modulation of disease severity in cystic fibrosis transmembrane conductance regulator deficient mice by a secondary genetic factor. *Nat Genet* 1996; **12**: 280–287.

16. Garred P, Madsen HO, Hofmann B, Svejgaard A. Increased frequency of homozygosity of abnormal mannan-binding-protein alleles in patients with suspected immunodeficiency. *Lancet* 1995; **346**: 941–943.

17. Garred P, Pressler T, Madsen HO *et al*. Association of mannose-binding lectin gene heterogeneity with severity of lung disease and survival in cystic fibrosis. *J Clin Invest* 1999; **104**: 431–437.

18. Mekus N, Ballmann M, Bronsveld I, Bijman J, Veeze H, Tummler B. Categories of ΔF508 homozygous cystic fibrosis twin and sibling pairs with distinct phenotypic characteristics. *Twin Res* 2000; **3**: 277–293.

19. Abdul WA, Al Thani G, Dawod ST, Kambouris M, Al Hamed M. Heterogeneity of the cystic fibrosis phenotype in a large kindred family in Qatar with cystic fibrosis mutation (I1234V). *J Trop Pediatr* 2001; **47**: 110–112.

20. Kosorok M, Zeng L, West S *et al*. Acceleration of lung disease in children with cystic fibrosis after *Pseudomonas aeruginosa* acquisition. *Pediatr Pulmonol* 2001; **32**: 277–287.

21. Hiatt PW, Grace SC, Kozinetz CA *et al*. Effects of viral lower respiratory tract infection on lung function in infants with cystic fibrosis. *Pediatrics* 1999; **103**: 619–626.

22. Dodge JA. Nutritional requirements in cystic fibrosis: a review. *J Pediatr Gastroenterol Nutr* 1988; **7**: S8–S11.

23. Bell SC, Bowerman AR, Davies CA, Campbell IA, Shale DJ, Elborn JS. Nutrition in adults with cystic fibrosis. *Clin Nutr* 1998; **17**: 211–215.

24. Ranganathan SC, Dezateux C, Bush A *et al*. Airway function in infants newly diagnosed with cystic fibrosis. *Lancet* 2001; **358**: 1964–1965.

25. Kerem E, Corey M, Bat-Sheva K *et al*. The relationship between genotype and phenotype in cystic fibrosis – analysis of the most common mutation (ΔF508). *N Engl J Med* 1990; **323**: 1517–1522.

26. Choudari CP, Lehman GA, Sherman S. Pancreatitis and cystic fibrosis gene mutations. *Gastroenterol Clin North Am* 1999; **28**: 543–549.

27. Wallis C. Diagnosing cystic fibrosis: blood, sweat, and tears. *Arch Dis Child* 1997; **76**: 85–88.

28. Dork T, Dworniczak B, Aulehla-Scholz C *et al*. Distinct spectrum of CFTR gene mutations in congenital absence of vas deferens. *Hum Genet* 1997; **100**: 365–377.

29. Dohle GR, Veeze HJ, Overbeek SE *et al*. The complex relationships between cystic fibrosis and congenital bilateral absence of the vas deferens: clinical, electrophysiological and genetic data. *Hum Reprod* 1999; **14**: 371–374.

30. Girodon E, Cazeneuve C, Lebargy F *et al*. CFTR gene mutations in adults with disseminated bronchiectasis. *Eur J Hum Genet* 1997; **5**: 149–155.

31. Milla C. Allergic bronchopulmonary aspergillosis and cystic fibrosis. *Pediatr Pulmonol* 1999; **27**: 71–73.

32. Miller P, Hamosh A, Macek M *et al.* Cystic fibrosis transmembrane conductance regulator (CFTR) gene mutations in allergic bronchopulmonary aspergillosis. *Am J Hum Genet* 1996; **59**: 45-51.

33. Sharer N, Schwartz M, Malone G *et al.* Mutations of the cystic fibrosis gene in patients with chronic pancreatitis. *N Engl J Med* 1998; **339**: 645–652.

34. Rosenstein BJ, Cutting GR. The diagnosis of cystic fibrosis: a consensus statement. Cystic Fibrosis Foundation Consensus Panel. *J Pediatr* 1998; **132**: 589–595.

35. Rosenstein BJ. Cystic fibrosis diagnosis: new dilemmas for an old disorder. *Pediatr Pulmonol* 2002; **33**: 83–84.

36. World Health Organization. *Classification of Cystic Fibrosis and Related Disorders* (WHO/ICF(M)A/ECFS/ECFTN). Geneva: WHO, 2000.

37. Bush A, Wallis C. Time to think again: cystic fibrosis is not an 'all or nothing' disease. *Pediatr Pulmonol* 2000; **30**: 139–144.

A. George F. Davidson Maggie McIlwaine

4

Positive expiratory pressure (PEP) masks, flutter devices and other mechanical aids to physiotherapy in cystic fibrosis

Physiotherapy, consisting of airway clearance techniques and exercise, is an integral part of the treatment of cystic fibrosis (CF). The goals of airway clearance techniques in CF are to remove tenacious airway secretions and decrease proteolytic activity in the airway, improve ventilation, reduce airway resistance and correct ventilation-perfusion mismatch. Long-term goals also include maintenance of normal chest mobility and posture, strengthening and conditioning of respiratory muscles, improving exercise tolerance, and improving self-esteem.[1]

In the past, the most commonly used airway clearance technique for CF was a combination of postural drainage and percussion administered by a caregiver, and often referred to as 'conventional chest physiotherapy'. Regular use of postural drainage and percussion improves pulmonary function in CF patients in the short-term[2] and slows deterioration in the long-term.[3,4]

The need for independence for older CF patients, high rates of non-compliance, and problems such as aspiration during postural drainage and percussion in CF patients with gastro-oesophageal reflux[5] have led to a search for alternative methods of airway clearance. Although a modified form of postural drainage and percussion can be performed independently using a mechanical percussor, these devices tend to be cumbersome and, in general, have fallen into disuse. Independence is now more readily achieved by replacing postural drainage and percussion with one of the newer airway

Prof. A. George F. Davidson BSc MD FRCPC[1,2] (for correspondence)

Ms Maggie McIlwaine MCSP CPA[2,3]

[1]Professor, Department of Pediatrics, University of British Columbia, Vancouver, Canada
[2]Cystic Fibrosis Clinic, British Columbia Children's Hospital, Vancouver, Canada
[3]Physiotherapy Department, British Columbia Children's Hospital, Vancouver, Canada

clearance techniques. However, caution must be used in selecting an airway clearance technique as not all the newer techniques or their variants have been proven to be clinically effective or to have advantages over postural drainage and percussion.

An increasing number of airway clearance techniques are now available based on a variety of physiological and physical principles. Each is usually performed as the sole airway clearance technique for the individual CF patient. In an attempt to standardize the techniques used, the International Physiotherapy (CF) Group and the International Cystic Fibrosis (Mucoviscidosis) Association have published guidelines for their performance.[6] Active cycle of breathing and autogenic drainage utilize expiratory airflow to mobilize secretions and do not rely on mechanical devices. However, PEP, high pressure PEP, flutter and high frequency chest-wall oscillation all require the use of mechanical devices for their performance. These mechanical aids and devices and their associated airway clearance techniques will be reviewed.

POSITIVE EXPIRATORY PRESSURE (PEP) MASK THERAPY

HISTORICAL AND THEORETICAL BACKGROUND

Positive expiratory pressure (PEP) was initially used postoperatively to re-inflate collapsed parts of the lungs by increasing collateral ventilation.[7] It was also found to have a secretion removal effect. In Denmark, Falk et al.[8] combined PEP with forced expiration (huffing) and coughing to mobilize and expectorate secretions, thus developing the PEP technique for CF, which was introduced in 1984.

The use of PEP in CF is based on the premise that retained secretions in the airways cause obstruction leading to impaired ventilation especially in the lung periphery and that methods to re-expand obstructed lung units are needed in order to mobilize secretions from the small airways. Once secretions are mobilized, airway collapse during expiration must be prevented in order to facilitate their clearance by expiratory airflow.

The physiological theories upon which the PEP technique is based suggest that PEP breathing increases collateral ventilation thus allowing air to 'get behind' the obstruction.[9] PEP may also influence the collateral time constant such that more air enters the collateral channels during inspiration than escapes during expiration, thus promoting a more even distribution of ventilation.[9] Groth et al.[10] have also demonstrated that functional residual capacity (FRC) is increased during tidal volume breathing using the PEP. The intraluminal positive pressure created by PEP during expiration prevents collapse of unstable airways due to an airflow-related decrease in intraluminal pressure (Bernoulli effect), and allows clearance of secretions to the larger airways. To complete the cycle, it is necessary to use forced expirations (without the mask) to mobilize secretions from the larger airways to where they may be effectively coughed-up and expectorated.

For PEP to be effective, a closed system is required throughout the 2 min breathing cycle in order to maintain positive end-expiratory pressure. This is best accomplished by means of a mask. It may be achieved using a mouthpiece, but this introduces the risk of artifact in which the pressure measured is oral and not airway.

TECHNIQUE AND EQUIPMENT

The original standard PEP airway clearance technique uses the Astra-Meditec system (Fig. 1). This system consists of a face mask and a one-way valve to which a flow-sensitive resistor is attached at the expiratory orifice, producing a positive pressure within the airways of 10–20 cmH$_2$O during expiration. A manometer can be inserted just proximal to the expiratory resistor to monitor the PEP pressure. The diameter of the resistor used for treatment is determined for each individual patient (1.5–3.0 mm). The exact counter pressure required to give the correct PEP level is not only determined by the size of the resistor but also by the patient's expiratory flow which varies from one individual to another. The size of resistor selected should be that at which the patient can maintain a steady PEP of 10–20 cmH$_2$O for 2 min of tidal volume breathing without exertion and with only slightly active expirations. Forceful and complete expiration is avoided, as it would only decrease lung volume.

The technique is performed in a sitting position with arms resting on a table. Each treatment cycle consists of 10–15 tidal volume breaths through the mask followed by forced expiratory manoeuvres consisting of huffing, interspersed with relaxed diaphragmatic breathing with the mask removed. The entire cycle is repeated five or six times or until as much sputum is cleared as possible.[8]

Bronchodilators can be delivered through the inspiratory port of the PEP system during the airway clearance technique, leading to enhanced efficacy[17] and time savings.

RESEARCH AND EVIDENCE OF EFFICACY OF THE PEP MASK TECHNIQUE

The largest number of studies reported in the literature on airway clearance techniques in CF relate to the PEP mask technique. No advantage has been

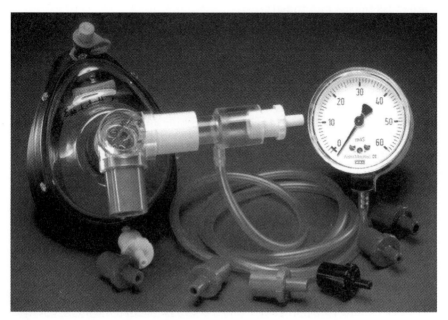

Fig. 1 Astra-Meditec PEP mask system.

shown in performing PEP in postural drainage positions.[8] In 1991, Mahlmmeister et al.[11] reviewed 38 studies comparing PEP to other techniques. The outcomes in the vast majority of these studies favoured PEP. Hofmeyer et al.[12] and Falk et al.[8] both attempted to compare PEP with the active cycle of breathing technique. These studies were very short-term with few patients and the two groups reported opposing results. Davidson et al.,[13] in a longer cross-over study comparing PEP with autogenic drainage and postural drainage and percussion in CF, reported both PEP and autogenic drainage to be equally as effective as postural drainage and percussion in maintaining pulmonary function. Two recent 1-year trials conducted in Canada have compared PEP with postural drainage and percussion. In the first study, performed on CF children,[14] a significant improvement in FVC and FEV_1 was found in the PEP group. In the second study on CF adults,[15] PEP was found to be as effective as postural drainage and percussion in slowing the decline in pulmonary function. In an editorial[16] referring to the first study,[14] Coates noted: 'one can now prescribe...PEP mask...in CF, confident that it meets or exceeds the accepted gold standard for chest physiotherapy'.

ALTERNATIVE TYPES OF PEP DEVICES

Many PEP devices other than the Astra-Meditec system have been developed since the 1980s. However, all research on the clinical efficacy of PEP has been conducted using the Astra-Meditec PEP device. Therefore, in assessing these newer devices, it is only possible to note how they compare to the original, both in method of use and with respect to achieving the same physiological and therapeutic effect. Evaluation of clinical efficacy of these newer devices at present can only be presumptive.

Face-mask versus mouthpiece

Therapists or patients sometimes substitute a mouthpiece for the face-mask, even when using the original Astra-Meditec system. However, this introduces the risk of artefact – if the cheeks are allowed to bulge, the expiratory pressure reading is the mouth pressure, which will be different from that in the intraluminal airway. If using a mouthpiece, nose-clips should also be used and cheeks kept flat. It is also more difficult with a mouthpiece to ensure that lung volumes are kept up throughout the whole of the airway clearance technique cycle of inhalation and exhalation because the patient's lips may not maintain the seal around the mouthpiece at the end of expiration.

TheraPEP

One of the newer PEP devices is the TheraPEP (Fig. 2). Usually, the device comes with a mouthpiece (but should be used with a face-mask) which is combined with a one-way valve and a selection of different sized expiratory orifices. A monitoring device is attached allowing feedback to keep the expiratory pressure between 10–20 cmH_2O. The pressure device is flow-dependent and, therefore, should achieve the same physiological effect as the Astra-Meditec mask system, provided care is taken when training the patient to ensure that the patient does not alter the size of breath to maintain the right pressures on the manometer, and instead achieves this by adjusting the size of

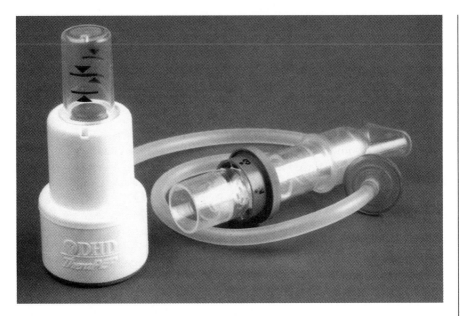

Fig. 2 TheraPEP.

the expiratory orifice. As is the case for the Astra-Meditec system, the aim is to maintain an expiratory pressure of between 10–20 cmH$_2$O while breathing at tidal volume with only slightly active expirations. The TheraPEP should be used exactly as recommended for the PEP technique, and combined with huffing and coughing.

PariPEP
The PariPEP is another flow-dependent PEP device, in this case designed to sit on top of a 'Pari' nebulizer. It consists of a one-way valve and different size expiratory orifices and a port to which a manometer or oxygen tubing can be attached. The primary purpose of the PariPEP is to maintain a positive expiratory pressure while delivering nebulized medications such as ventolin. By splinting the airways open using a PEP device, it is believed that medication can be delivered further down the respiratory tract.[17] If the primary purpose of using the PariPEP is for improved delivery of medications, then normal tidal breathing through the mouthpiece is sufficient to achieve that aim. However, in CF the PariPEP is often used to achieve airway clearance as well as delivery of medications. In this case, the method of using the PariPEP needs to be the same as for the PEP mask technique.

Threshold devices
Threshold devices are PEP systems that use a (pressure) threshold resistor. These usually consist of a one-way spring valve, which can be adjusted to different water pressures between 5–25 cmH$_2$O. These are not flow-dependant valves and, therefore, the system operates independently of expiratory airflow. While PEP systems based on this type of device maintain a positive expiratory pressure which can splint the airways open, the expiratory flow may not be

sufficient to mobilize secretions; hence, these devices can not be recommended for airway clearance.

HIGH PRESSURE PEP THERAPY

HISTORICAL AND THEORETICAL BACKGROUND

This airway clearance technique was developed in Austria upon a different premise to that of the 'standard' or 'low pressure' PEP. For high pressure PEP, it is postulated that forced expiration against a marked resistive load will 'squeeze' air from hyperinflated into obstructed and atelectatic lung units. The high expiratory pressure resistance causes a completely homogenized slow expiratory evacuation of all lung units, regardless of whether thay are distal to obstructed or bronchiectatic airways. When monitored by a flow-volume curve, this effect is expressed as a plateau formation in the expiratory tracing. As the treatment cycle proceeds, the loss of lung volume effects a decrease of static-elastic recoil pressure to such an extent that the plateau formation cannot be maintained and the equal pressure point previously arrested at the resistor moves upstream towards the bronchial periphery. The terminal phase of the expiratory high pressure PEP manoeuvre effects dynamic compression of all bronchial airways. With high pressure PEP there is a reduced expiratory airflow velocity when compared to the standard PEP mask technique. The proponents of high pressure PEP believe this is counterbalanced by the effects of dynamic expiratory bronchial compression.

TECHNIQUE

The high pressure PEP technique[18] uses the same system (*i.e.* the Astra-Meditec mask) as for regular PEP, but with a higher pressure expiratory resistor and different technique. The resistance is determined individually for each patient on the basis of maximal homogenisation in the expiratory behaviour of the different lung units as determined by the shape of the flow-volume curve.[18] The forced expiratory manoeuvres usually create an expiratory pressure between 40–100 cmH_2O depending on lung size, expiratory muscle force, training, airway wall stability and stage of the pulmonary disease.

The technique is performed in a sitting position, while leaning into the mask. The treatment cycle includes 8–10 tidal volume breaths with a slight emphasis on expiration followed by a full forced expiratory manoeuvre through the mask to mobilize and transport secretions.. After coughing and expectoration, the patient repeats the cycle until maximum clearance of secretions is achieved. No adverse effects have been reported, although some patients find it too uncomfortable to huff against the high positive pressure. The developers of this technique emphasize that the method should be used only in specialized centres capable of selecting and controlling the PEP-mask resistance and monitoring the patient's technique.

RESEARCH AND EVIDENCE OF EFFICACY OF HIGH PRESSURE PEP

Studies on the use of high pressure PEP have been very limited and only reported from one centre, where the efficacy of the technique has been documented with regard to removal of airway secretions.[18,19] Further studies, including clinical outcome studies over a longer term and reports from other CF centres, need to be performed in order to validate the high pressure PEP technique for general use.

OSCILLATING POSITIVE EXPIRATORY PRESSURE AND THE FLUTTER DEVICE VRP₁

HISTORICAL AND THEORETICAL BACKGROUND

In the late 1980s, a PEP device which also produced oscillations in expiratory pressure and intermittent acceleration of the expiratory airflow, was developed in Switzerland. This device, the Flutter VRP_1 (Fig. 3), was first introduced to facilitate the removal of secretions from the airways in patients with COPD and cystic fibrosis. Since its introduction, several other oscillating PEP devices have been developed such as the RC Cornet and the Acapella.

The rationale upon which Flutter VRP_1 is based is that the positive pressure prevents the early collapse that can occur in unstable bronchial airways and increases the diameter of the airways up to the peripheral bronchioles, while the oscillations facilitate the clearance of mucus.[20] The oscillations can be 'tuned' to the patient's own lung resonance frequency, thereby inducing maximal vibrations of the bronchial walls and promoting clearance of the small airways.[22] The proponents of this technique do not rely on collateral ventilation to open up obstructed lung units. Instead, to equalize ventilation, the patient is instructed to inhale and hold their breath for 2–3 s before starting expiration.

The Flutter VRP_1 (VarioRaw) is a pocket-sized, pipe-like device consisting of a mouthpiece connected to the bottom of a plastic cone which holds a steel ball, and a perforated cover. During expiration, the pressure of the exhaled air pushes the steel ball up the cone wall. This allows the air to escape and the

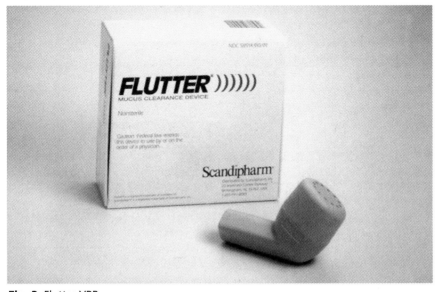

Fig. 3 Flutter VRP_1.

pressure to drop, whereupon the steel ball returns to its previous position and the cycle repeats. Endobronchial pressure pulses of between 10–25 cmH$_2$O and oscillations of between 6–26 Hz are generated during expiration through this device. The frequency of the oscillations can be modulated by adjusting the angle at which the Flutter is held to the mouth during expiration. The optimum position of the Flutter is one that creates a frequency that resonates with the individual's naturally occurring pulmonary resonance. This is usually between 8–16 Hz.

TECHNIQUE

While in a sitting position, the patient inhales deeply, holds their breath for 2–3 s, then exhales through the Flutter device, breathing out actively into the expiratory reserve volume. On exhalation, the patient may need to tilt the Flutter device up or down slightly by a few degrees until maximum vibrations are felt within their airways ('tuning to the resonance frequency of the lungs'). At the end of 10–12 breaths through the Flutter, the patient performs 1 or 2 huffs (also through the Flutter) to promote mobilization of more central secretions, followed by a cough.

RESEARCH AND EVIDENCE OF EFFICACY OF FLUTTER (VRP$_1$)

Many studies have been conducted relating to the Flutter VRP$_1$. Dasgupta, King and App[21,23,24] demonstrated a decrease in the spinnability and visco-elastic properties of mucus when oscillation is applied and showed that oscillations of expiratory airflow can alter the physical properties of airway secretions by mechanically rupturing the rigid mucous gel, hence decreasing viscosity.[21] It has been suggested that these phenomena together with the oscillations in airflow and pressure lead to mobilization and removal of secretions during the use of oscillating PEP.

Clinical studies of efficacy have in general been short-term and with varying results. In an influential short-term clinical study, Konstan et al.[25] found that the amount of sputum expectorated by patients using the Flutter was more than 3 times that expectorated after either voluntary cough or 1 min of percussion in each of 11 PD positions. In another study when Flutter was compared to the active cycle of breathing technique (ACBT) over a 2-day period, significantly more sputum was cleared with ACBT than by the Flutter.[26]

The only published study reporting long-term effects of using the Flutter VRP$_1$ as the sole device for airway clearance, found the Flutter technique to have significant deleterious effects on the pulmonary function of patients with cystic fibrosis.[27] In this study, Flutter was performed as recommended by Konstan et al.,[25] i.e. the standard method for North America which requires the patient to exhale into their expiratory reserve volume (ERV). The authors of this study hypothesized that the negative effects found with the Flutter were due to exhaling into the ERV, since this would cause no end-expiratory positive pressure to be maintained, and hence the airways would not be splinted open during the late expiratory phase of breathing. The work of Schibler and Kraemer appears to support this suggestion, since they have shown on flow volume and pressure volume curves that intrabronchial pressure falls when breathing at the ERV level through the Flutter.[28] It may be that breathing at these low lung volumes with oscillating positive pressures and airway vibration leads to some airway closure resulting in increased air trapping and a decrease in FVC. The Bernoulli effect of airflow causing a fall in the intra-airway pressure may enhance such collapse of airways. This study shows that not only is the type of medical device used in a study important, but also the prescribed method of using the device. The manufacturers of the Flutter VRP$_1$ now recommend that patients should only exhale slightly into their expiratory reserve volume through the device, but no studies have been performed to validate this new method of using the Flutter. It is also not known whether the airway vibrations caused by the device may in the long-term have deleterious effects on airway stability.

ALTERNATIVE TYPES OF OSCILLATING POSITIVE EXPIRATORY PRESSURE DEVICES

RC-CORNET

The RC-Cornet consists of a mouthpiece, a rubber hose that is encased in a bent plastic tube and a sound damper (Fig. 4). As the patient exhales through the RC-Cornet, the hose pressure increases and the hose buckles at the bend in the outer tube. At a critical pressure (between 5–20 cmH$_2$O), the hose straightens against the wall of the tube, air escapes and the end of the hose turns outwards. The hose then bends, pressure builds up and the process is repeated, providing an oscillation effect with defined fluctuations in pressure and flow.

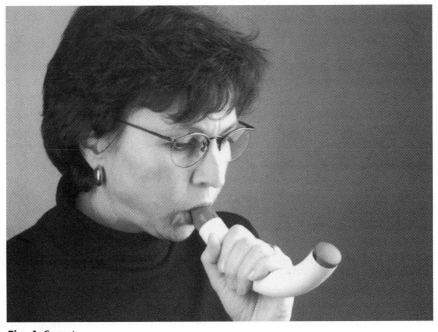

Fig. 4 Cornet.

The rationale for the RC-Cornet is the same as for the Flutter. The proponents of this device believe the RC-Cornet offers several advantages over the Flutter VRP$_1$. In the case of the Flutter, both pressure and flow-rate are reduced during exhalation, whilst using the RC-Cornet, pressure and flow-rate are kept more or less constant up to the end of the exhalation period. Blackney et al.[29] showed the RC-Cornet generated lower peak pressures, lower frequencies and greater amplitude when compared to the Flutter. The method of using the RC-Cornet is similar to the Flutter. Patients are also instructed to exhale into their ERV through the RC-Cornet, which may have detrimental effects, as discussed previously for the Flutter VRP$_1$.

ACAPELLA

The Acapella is the newest oscillatory PEP device on the market. It consists of a mouthpiece (it may also be used with a face-mask) and a plastic cone-shaped cylinder which contains a one-way inspiratory valve and is divided horizontally in half to allow the patient to inhale as well as exhale through the device. Exhalation is through a vibratory rocker assembly consisting of a magnet and a counterweighted plug. This creates oscillations of between 0–30 Hz while maintaining a positive pressure throughout the exhalation. The Acapella comes in two sizes, one for patients with expiratory flows of > 15 l/min and one for flows of < 15 l/min as measured during 3 s of expiration through the device. Pressure, frequency and flow rates are adjusted by turning a dial at the end of the cylinder. The expiratory pressure generated through the Acapella is between 10–20 cmH$_2$O. Pressure may be monitored by inserting a pressure gauge between the cylinder and mouthpiece.

The instructions given to the patient are similar to those for a patient using a PEP mask, with the exception that there is a 3 s breath hold on inspiration. Expiration is to functional residual capacity only. This is the only oscillating PEP device allowing inhalation and exhalation through the device. The physiological basis of the Acapella is the same as for the PEP mask with the added feature of oscillation, which it is suggested, promotes loosening of secretions from the airway walls.

RESEARCH AND EVIDENCE OF EFFICACY

Dasgupta[30] reported that although both Flutter and RC-Cornet decreased the cohesiveness of mucus, the Flutter was significantly more effective. The long-term clinical effects of these devices have not been evaluated, and it is not possible to extrapolate their clinical efficacy from experience with PEP or Flutter. Therefore, neither device can be recommend for airway clearance in CF at this time.

HIGH FREQUENCY CHEST WALL OSCILLATION ('THE VEST')

HISTORICAL AND THEORETICAL BACKGROUND

Early experimental studies found an increased rate of mucus clearance and increased airflow after applying sharp compression pulses to the lower thorax

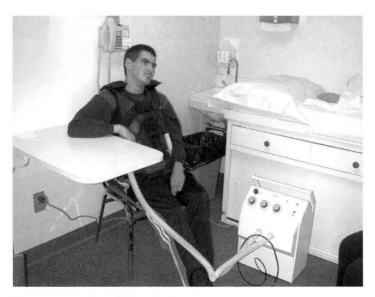

Fig. 5 High frequency chest wall oscillation vest.

of dogs via a piston pump and modified blood pressure cuff. In 1985, Gross *et al.*,[32] using a radio-tagged aerosol, oberved significant increases in mucus mobilization and peripheral airway clearance during high frequency chest wall oscillation. Several possible mechanisms of action have been proposed. The compression pulses are thought to produce transient cephalad airflow bias spikes in the airway comparable to a huffing manoeuver.[33] The shear forces associated with the oscillating airflow are thought to decrease visco-elasticity of mucus similar to that shown for oscillating PEP,[23] and to help loosen secretions from the airway walls.

In 1989, Warwick designed the first high frequency chest wall oscillation vest for human subjects. The device has undergone several design changes since its inception which affect the compression curve applied as well as the design of the vest itself. The most common model in use today is the ThAIRapy Bronchial Drainage System (American Biosystems Inc.; Fig. 5) which uses variable compression frequencies of between 5–25 Hz.

TECHNIQUE

The treatment session is usually performed in a sitting position. The vest, which is designed to fit over the entire thorax, has a port on either side of the front panel which connects via large bore tubing to the air pulse generator. The vest inflates against the patient's chest wall at a set pressure, usually 5 cmH$_2$O, then small pulses of air are rapidly injected and withdrawn. The pulses cause the vest to inflate and deflate against the thorax of the patient, creating a vibratory or 'oscillatory' motion. Usually three different fequencies are used between 5–25 Hz for a 5 min period. Recently, the manufacturer has advised patients that it is only necessary to use one frequency but for a longer duration, interupted by huffing and coughing.

RESEARCH AND EVIDENCE OF EFFICACY

A number of studies have been performed on high frequency chest wall oscillation, including short-term clinical studies. In general, these suggest that the vest is as effective as other commonly used airway clearance techniques. In one such study, Braggion *et al.* found high frequency chest wall oscillation, PEP and postural drainage and percussion mobilized significantly greater amounts of sputum in CF patients compared to no treatment.[34] In another short-term study, Kluft[35] showed high frequency chest wall oscillation produced significantly more sputum in CF patients when compared to postural drainage and percussion. However, to date, there have been no reports of long-term comparative trials with high frequency chest wall oscillation.

As well as the lack of long-term clinical outcome information, the size and cost (over US$16,000) of the high frequency chest wall oscillation equipment is an obstacle to its use. There may be specific situations where the device is useful, such as for very ill patients who lack the strength to perform other airway clearance techniques, or in patients who for some other reason are unable to perform other airway clearance techniques.

BIPOLAR POSITIVE AIRWAY PRESSURE (BiPAP)

Bipolar positive airway pressure may be used to help support the CF patient who has end-stage pulmonary disease, while awaiting lung transplant. At this stage, physiotherapy is very tiring and the patient may not be able to tolerate an airway clearance technique. While bipolar positive airway pressure is not primarily designed as an airway clearance technique device, it is possible to modify the bipolar positive airway pressure settings from a high inspiratory and low expiratory pressure to a low inspiratory and high expiratory pressure for short periods of time. In this mode, the bipolar positive airway pressure machine functions similarly to a PEP mask device. Huffing or assisted huffing and coughing may then be performed with or without the bipolar positive airway pressure machine.

ADJUNCTIVE THERAPIES

Bronchodilators, inhaled steriods and DNase are often given in combination with an airway clearance technique to enhance its effectiveness. Exercise also complements airway clearance techniques, inducing a significant increase in sputum production.[4] Regular exercise, especially running and swimming, can also improve respiratory muscle function, cardiorespiratory conditioning, muscle strength, exercise tolerance, sense of well-being, and self-image.[36] Any physical exercise prescription for children with pulmonary disease should include stretching, strengthening and an aerobic component.

CHOOSING AN AIRWAY CLEARANCE TECHNIQUE FOR YOUR PATIENT

The CF patient and CF family should incorporate airway clearance techniques, exercise, and any adjunctive drug therapy into their life-style and develop a consistent daily routine. This is more likely to occur if physiotherapy is commenced as soon after diagnosis as possible, and then regularly reviewed in the CF clinic.

In babies and young toddlers who are unable to actively assist in performing treatments, postural drainage and percussion is the usual airway clearance technique used. However, the PEP mask can also be used for infants if the care-giver is taught to hold the PEP mask over the infant's face, while the infant sits on the care-giver's lap. It is not possible to include huffing at this age, but the proponents of this method maintain that breathing through the PEP mask is the most important part of this airway clearance technique. Vests for the high frequency chest wall oscillation technique are also available to fit a child as young as 2 years of age. As the toddler becomes more actively involved in treatment, blowing games, huffing and exercise in the form of playful activities should be introduced. By the age of 4–6 years, the child should be actively participating in their therapy.

After the age of 4 or 5 years of age, the child previously on postural drainage and percussion is usually ready for another airway clearance technique to be introduced. The technique chosen will depend on the individual and the situation. Selection criteria will depend on:

1. Airway disease state, *i.e.* obstruction, restriction, hyper-reactivity, instability.

2. Subjective and objective evaluation, *i.e.* mucus production, cough, chest radiographs, pulmonary function, auscultation, activity level, feeling of well-being.

3. Other factors, *i.e.* age, compliance, co-operation, culture, family dynamics, techniques presently being used, and skill level.

The PEP mask or high pressure PEP are particularly useful for patients who have difficulty clearing secretions because of unstable airways. The PEP mask can also deliver bronchodilators more effectively and decrease treatment time. The high frequency chest wall oscillation vest may also be uniquely useful for the CF patient who, for whatever reason, is unable to learn or perform other airway clearance techniques. It is important that, whatever technique is chosen for a patient, it be taught by an experienced physiotherapist, knowledgable in all airway clearance techniques who will be able to optimise the technique to suit the individual's needs.

Key points for clinical practice

- Physiotherapy, consisting of airway clearance techniques and exercise, is a critical component of care for patients with cystic fibrosis and should be instituted at diagnosis.

- Regular daily use of a clinically proven airway clearance technique has been shown to improve pulmonary function in cystic fibrosis patients in the short-term and to minimize deterioration in the long-term.

Key points for clinical practice (continued)

- The 'standard' airway clearance technique in common use has been postural drainage and percussion performed by a care-giver. Mechanical percussors for postural drainage and percussion have been used in an attempt to promote independance for older patients, but tend to be cumbersome and have fallen into disuse.

- Other, newer, airway clearance techniques can be performed by the cystic fibrosis patient alone, allowing greater independence.

- Airway clearance techniques in current use include postural drainage and percussion, active cycle of breathing, autogenic drainage, positive expiratory pressure (PEP), high pressure PEP, oscillating PEP and high frequency chest wall oscillation. Different airway clearance techniques are based upon different physiological and physical principles and premises.

- PEP, high pressure PEP, oscillating PEP and high frequency chest wall oscillation airway clearance techniques require the use of mechanical aids or devices designed specifically for that airway clearance technique.

- The physiological and clinical effects achieved using an airway clearance device are dependent on adherence to the specific airway clearance technique for which that device was developed.

- Results obtained with an airway clearance technique in which an alternative or modified technique or device is used, may not be the same as those obtained with the original technique or device.

- Of the devices for airway clearance in current use, only the (Astra-Meditec) PEP mask and its associated airway clearance technique has been proven by long-term clinical trials to be equal or superior to postural drainage and percussion.

- Other, currently used airway clearance technique devices have not yet been proven to have long-term clinical benefit for the cystic fibrosis patient. Some airway clearance techniques and devices currently promoted may have deleterious effects on the cystic fibrosis patient.

- Factors that affect choice of airway clearance technique include, age, disease state, airway stability and reactivity, social and cultural influences.

References

1. Schoni MH. Autogenic drainage: a modern approach to physiotherapy in cystic fibrosis. *J R Soc Med* 1989; **82 (Suppl 16)**: 1792–1797.
2. Desmond KJ, Schwenk WF, Thomas E, Beaudry PH, Coates AL. Immediate and long-term effects of chest physiotherapy in patients with cystic fibrosis. *J Pediatr* 1983; **103**: 538–542.

3. Reisman JJ, Rivington-Law B, Corey M *et al.* Role of conventional physiotherapy in cystic fibrosis. *J Pediatr* 1988; **113**: 632–636.

4. Thomas J, Cook DJ, Brooks D. Chest physical therapy management of patients with cystic fibrosis. *Am J Respir Crit Care Med* 1995; **151**: 846–850.

5. Button BM, Heine RG, Catto-Smith AG, Pheland PD, Olinsky A. Postural drainage in infants: to tip or not to tip, that is the question. *Pediatr Pulmonol* 1985; **Suppl 12**: 108–109.

6. International Cystic Fibrosis Physiotherapy Group. *Physiotherapy in the Treatment of Cystic Fibrosis*, (2nd edn in Press).International CF (Mucoviscidosis) Association, 1995.

7. Menkes HA, Traystman RJ. Collateral ventilation. *Am Rev Respir Dis* 1977; **116**: 287–309.

8. Falk M, Kelstrup M, Anderson JB. Improving the ketchup bottle method with positive expiratory pressure. A controlled study in patients with cystic fibrosis. *Eur J Respir Dis* 1984; **63**: 423–432.

9. Anderson JB, Qvist J, Kann T. Recruiting collapsed lung through collateral channels with positive end-expiratory pressure. *Scand J Respir Dis* 1979; **60**: 260–266.

10. Groth S, Stafanger G, Durkson H, Anderson JB, Falk M, Kelstrup M. Positive expiratory pressure (PEP-mask) physiotherapy improves ventilation and reduces volume of trapped gas in cystic fibrosis. *Clin Respir Physiol* 1985; **21**: 339–343.

11. Mahlmeister MJ, Fink JB, Hoffman GL, Fifer LF. Positive expiratory pressure mask therapy: theoretical and practical considerations and a review of the literature. *Respir Care* 1991; **36**: 1218–1229.

12. Hofmeyr JL, Webber BA, Hodson ME. Evaluation of positive expiratory pressure as an adjunct to chest physiotherapy in the treatment of cystic fibrosis. *Thorax* 1986; **41**: 951–954.

13. Davidson AGF, McIlwaine PM, Wong LTK, Nakielna EM, Pirie GE. A comparative trial of positive expiratory pressure, autogenic drainage and conventional percussion and drainage techniques. *Pediatr Pulmonol* 1988; **Suppl 2**: 137.

14. McIlwaine PM, Wong LTK, Peacock D, Davidson AGF. Long-term comparative trial of conventional postural drainage and percussion versus positive expiratory pressure physiotherapy in the treatment of cystic fibrosis. *J Pediatr* 1997; **131**: 570–574.

15. Gaskin L. Long-term trial of conventional postural drainage and percussion versus positive expiratory pressure. *Pediatr Pulmonol* 2000; **Suppl 17**: 322

16. Coates AL. Chest physiotherapy in cystic fibrosis: spare the hand and spoil the cough?. *J Pediatr* 1997; **131**: 506–508.

17. Christensen EF, Norregaard O. Inhaled beta$_2$ agonist and positive expiratory pressure in bronchial asthma. Influence on airway resistance and functional residual capacity. *Chest* 1993; **104**: 1108–1113

18. Oberwaldner B. Forced expirations against a variable resistance: a new chest physiotherapy method in cystic fibrosis. *Pediatr Pulmonol* 1986; **Suppl 2**: 358–367.

19. Pfleger A, Theibl B, Oberwaldner B, Zach MS. Self-administered chest physiotherapy in cystic fibrosis: a comparative study of high-pressure PEP and autogenic drainage. *Lung* 1992; **170**: 323–330.

20. Althaus P. The bronchial hygiene assisted by the Flutter VRP$_1$. *Eur Respir J* 1989; **Suppl 8**: 2,693.

21. Dasgupta B, App EM, King M. Effects of the Flutter device and airflow oscillations on spinnability of cystic fibrosis sputum. *Am J Respir Crit Care Med* 1996; **153**: A69.

22. Lindeman H. The value of physical therapy with VRPI Destin (Flutter). *Pneumologie* 1992; **46**: 626–630.

23. Dasgupta B, Brown NE, King M. Effects of sputum oscillations and rhDNase *in vitro*: a combined approach to treat cystic fibrosis lung disease. *Pediatr Pulmonol* 1998; **26**: 250–255.

24. App EM. Sputum rheology changes in cystic fibrosis lung disease following two different types of physiotherapy: Flutter vs autogenic drainage. *Chest* 1998; **114**: 171–177.

25. Konstan MW, Stern RC, Doershuk CF, Matthews LW. Efficacy of the Flutter device for airway mucus clearance in patients with cystic fibrosis. *J Pediatr* 1994; **124**: 689–693.

26. Pryor JA, Webber BA, Hodson ME, Warner JO. The Flutter VRP$_1$ as an adjunct to chest physiotherapy in cystic fibrosis. *Respir Med* 1994; **88**: 677–681.

27. McIlwaine M, Wong LTK, Peacock D, Davidson AGF. Long-term comparative trial of positive expiratory pressure (PEP) versus oscillating positive expiratory pressure (Flutter) in the treatment of cystic fibrosis. *J Pediatr* 2001; **138**: 845–850.

28. Schibler A, Kraemer R. *Flutter® Handbook*. Scandipharm Inc., 1995; 19.

29. Blackney DA, Chipps B. Comparison of airway pressure and oscillation frequency of four airway clearance devices. *Pediatr Pulmonol* 1998; **Suppl 16**: A430.

30. Dasgupta B, Nakamura S, App EM, King M. Comparative evaluation of the Flutter and the Cornet in improving the cohesiveness of cystic fibrosis sputum. *Pediatr Pulmonol* 1997; **Suppl 14**: 300.

31. King M, Phillips DM, Gross D, Varitian V, Chang HK, Zidulka A. Enhanced tracheal mucus clearance with high frequency chest wall compression. *Am Rev Respir Dis* 1983; **128**: 511–515.

32. Gross D, Zidulka A, O'Brien C *et al*. Peripheral mucociliary clearance with high frequency chest wall compression. *J Appl Physiol* 1985; **58**: 1157–1163.

33. Hansen LG, Warwick WJ. High-frequency chest compression system to aid in clearance of mucus from the lung. *Biomed Instrum Technol* 1990; **24**: 289–294.

34. Braggion C, Cappelletti LM, Cornacchia M, Zanolla L, Mastella G. Short-term effects of three chest physiotherapy regimens in patients hospitalized for pulmonary exacerbations of cystic fibrosis: a cross-over randomized study. *Pediatr Pulmonol* 1995; **19**: 16–22.

35. Kluft J, Beker L, Castagnino M, Gaiser J, Chaney H, Fink R. A comparison of bronchial drainage treatments in cystic fibrosis. *Pediatr Pulmonol* 1996; **22**: 271–274.

36. Cerny FJ, Pullano TP, Cropp GJA. Cardiorespiratory adaptations to exercise in cystic fibrosis. *Am Rev Respir Dis* 1982; **126**: 217–222.

J.H. Smith S.A. Kanagasundaram

5

Nitrous oxide in alleviating pain and anxiety during painful procedures in children

PROCEDURAL PAIN

Children can be exposed to painful medical procedures during an admission to hospital, a visit to the out-patient clinic, accident and emergency department or the family doctor. The procedure may be diagnostic and/or therapeutic, a solitary one-off event or part of an on-going management plan. Venous cannulation, bone marrow aspiration, lumbar puncture, removal of chest drain and dressings changes are some examples. The combination of a single or multiple procedures can not only be painful but separation from parents and being in a strange environment can also be anxiety provoking.[1]

Pain and anxiety levels related to individual procedures are influenced by a number of factors. Procedural factors such as invasiveness and duration will

---

Table 1 Properties of the ideal agent for painful procedures

- Analgesia
- Anxiolysis
- Predictable and rapid onset
- Rapid offset
- Amnesia
- Minimal side-effects
- Painless administration

Dr Jonathan H. Smith FRCA
Specialist Registrar in Anaesthesia

Dr Suchitra A. Kanagasundaram FRCA FANZCA (for correspondence)
Consultant Anaesthetist, The Whittington Hospital, Highgate Hill, London N19 5NF, UK
Tel +20 7288 5464; E-mail: skanagasundaram@aol.com

dictate the amount of tissue trauma caused. Patient factors such as previous pain experiences, current fear and anxiety levels, coping styles, cultural beliefs and prognosis will influence their response to the procedure. Other factors such as the attitudes and beliefs of parents and staff and the physical environment in which the procedure is performed all play a role in determining how the procedure is tolerated.[1]

APPROACH TO PROCEDURAL PAIN

Management of procedural pain includes alleviation of anxiety and pain to enable the procedure to be conducted with minimal distress to the child. This is best achieved using the technique of conscious sedation which is defined as: 'a technique in which the use of a drug or drugs produces a state of depression of the central nervous system enabling treatment to be carried out, but during which verbal contact with the patient is maintained throughout the period of sedation'.[2] An ideal sedative technique should produce a rapid and smooth onset of action and allow for control of the level of sedation in relation to the degree of stimulation from the procedure. The technique should also allow the child to recover rapidly to full alertness without rebound or emergence effects. A degree of amnesia is particularly beneficial for children requiring repeated painful procedures. The sedation technique must be safe and not contribute to any morbidity or mortality. In particular, it should be safe when used by surgeons and physicians as well as anaesthetists.

To ensure safety, The Royal College of Anaesthetists has published a document outlining 'safe sedation practice'.[2] Although relating to adult practice, the points raised are also relevant to paediatric procedures. As well as maintaining verbal contact throughout the procedure, the report recommends that the patient is assessed pre-procedure and monitored by a trained individual using at least pulse oximetry throughout the procedure. There should be facilities for the immediate administration of oxygen, and provision of head-down tilt of the trolley, and appropriate resuscitation equipment must be available until full recovery of the patient.[2]

The best way to ensure safe sedation is to have a trained member of staff present at all times whose sole responsibility is the administration of sedation and monitoring of the child. Most paediatric units now have treatment rooms in their respective wards which have appropriate monitoring facilities and properly trained staff.

IDEAL AGENTS FOR PAINFUL PROCEDURES

Various pharmacological agents have been used alone and in combination with varying degree of success.[1] The properties of an ideal agent for procedural pain include analgesia, anxiolysis, amnesia and minimal side-effects. The agent should also have a rapid and predictable onset with characteristics that allow early recovery and discharge. A painless route of administration is also important (Table 1).

Unfortunately none of the currently used agents meets all these criteria. The agents that are commonly used in children include benzodiazepines often in combination with an opioid, ketamine and chloral hydrate.[3–5] The benzodiazepines are frequently used for sedation, but their effects can be unpredictable and long-lasting. When used in combination with an opioid, there is an increased risk of respiratory depression, inadvertent loss of consciousness and subsequent loss of airway patency and protection.

Nitrous oxide, which possesses both sedative and analgesic effects with rapid onset and offset, is being used much more widely for painful procedures in the hospital setting.

NITROUS OXIDE (N$_2$O)

HISTORY OF NITROUS OXIDE

Joseph Priestley first isolated nitrous oxide in 1772 and in 1795 Humphry Davy described its analgesic properties.[6] At that time, N$_2$O was widely used as a recreational drug, its effects leading it to be described as 'laughing gas'. Horace Wells (an American dentist) first used nitrous oxide during the extraction of his own tooth in 1844.[6] In the present day, it is widely used as a component of balanced general anaesthesia and for analgesia during childbirth, by paramedics, and during painful procedures in hospitals.

PROPERTIES OF NITROUS OXIDE

Nitrous oxide is a sweet-smelling, colourless gas with a molecular weight of 44.01.[7] It is presented in blue cylinders with blue shoulders. Although non-flammable, nitrous oxide supports combustion, especially so when mixed with oxygen. When inhaled, nitrous oxide immediately starts to have an effect that peaks at 1–2 min. Once inhalation ceases, nitrous oxide is rapidly eliminated unchanged by the lungs.[7]

ANALGESIC AND ANAESTHETIC EFFECTS OF NITROUS OXIDE

Nitrous oxide is a powerful analgesic and a weak anaesthetic agent. It is claimed that 20–50% nitrous oxide in oxygen gives comparable pain relief to 15 mg of morphine or 100 mg of pethidine in adults.[8,9] The mechanism of analgesia is a complex combination of opioid and noradrenergic actions.[10] There may also be an action at NMDA receptors that influences post-injury hyperalgesia.[11]

Work on rats less than 3 weeks of age has shown that the noradrenergic neurones required for nitrous oxide mediated analgesia have not yet developed. As a 3-week-old rat is comparable in neurological development to a human toddler, it has been suggested that nitrous oxide may not exert its usual analgesic effects in this age group.[12]

If inhaled at concentrations above 70%, nitrous oxide begins to have an anaesthetic effect and a decreased level of consciousness will occur. This effect is greatly enhanced if other central nervous depressants are present. Complete surgical anaesthesia using nitrous oxide alone can only occur at supra-atmospheric pressures such as those found in a hyperbaric chamber, an unlikely setting for most routine painful procedures!

MODES OF DELIVERY

Nitrous oxide is widely used for analgesia and sedation during painful procedures in children (Table 2). There are two main routes of delivery, from a

Table 2 Painful procedures completed in children using nitrous oxide as analgesia

Venepuncture/venous cannulation[16,18,19,22,24,26]	Bone marrow aspiration[19]
Portacath flush[16]	Lumbar puncture[18,19,22]
Suture insertion/removal[16,18,19,25]	Nasal packing[19]
Drain removal[16,18]	Renal biopsy[19,23]
Change of dressing[16–19,22]	Lymph node biopsy[19]
Physiotherapy[17]	Bladder catheterisation[19]
Dental care[19]	Insertion of NG tube[16]
Orthopaedic traction adjustment[16–19]	Botulinum injections[16]
Change of plaster cast[17–19]	Pulmonary endoscopy[19]
Fracture manipulation[18–20,27]	Gastrointestinal endoscopy[21]
Removal of Ilizarov frame/K wires/skeletal pins[17–19]	Minor surgery (nail surgery, foreign body exploration, abscess drainage)[19,22]

pre-filled cylinder containing 50% oxygen and 50% nitrous oxide (Entonox®) or via a face-mask attached to a 'relative analgesia'(RA) machine that delivers a variable mixture of oxygen (30–100%) and nitrous oxide (0–70%) by continuous flow.

ENTONOX®

The 50:50 mix of nitrous oxide and oxygen known as Entonox® was first used as an analgesic during child-birth in 1961 and then adopted by the ambulance service in 1970.[13]

Physical properties of Entonox®

Entonox® is presented in cylinders that are blue with blue and white shoulders. As with pure nitrous oxide, Entonox® is a colourless, sweet-smelling gas that is non-flammable but strongly supports combustion.[7] At temperatures below –6°C, the nitrous oxide begins to separate out creating the possibility of delivering a hypoxic mixture. If this is a possibility, storing the cylinders horizontally for 24 h above 10°C, or warming at 10°C for 2 h and then completely inverting 3 times can ensure a homogenous mixture.[7]

Delivery of Entonox®

Entonox® is delivered through an on-demand valve that requires –2 to –5 cmH$_2$O of inspiratory effort to open. The gas mixture is then inhaled via a mouthpiece or one of a range of face-masks (Fig. 1). As the child holds the mask or mouthpiece in place themselves, the delivery apparatus will fall away from their face if excessive sedation occurs, hence terminating the flow of Entonox®.

Hypoxia is very rare whilst using Entonox® because there is the added safety of inhaling 50% oxygen throughout the whole procedure.

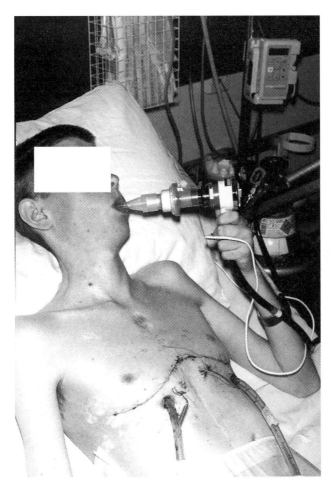

Fig. 1 Entonox® delivered through an on-demand valve and inhaled via a mouthpiece.

DELIVERY OF VARIABLE CONCENTRATIONS

Nitrous oxide can be administered at a variable concentration (0–70%) using a continuous flow device. The advantage is that, at a concentration of nitrous oxide within 50–70%, a plane of total analgesia can be reached.[14] The equipment for delivery of nitrous oxide at a variable concentration is similar to that used for sedation in dental surgeries. A combined flow meter for nitrous oxide and oxygen and a mixture control allow the delivery of a variable concentration of nitrous oxide (0–70%) while limiting the maximum concentration of nitrous oxide to 70% (Fig. 2). The equipment also consists of an antihypoxic device and a fail-safe delivery of 30% oxygen at all times. The unit is attached to a Bain circuit and mask for delivery of gases to the patient.

The delivery of concentrations of nitrous oxide greater than 50% demands close supervision so as to monitor the level of consciousness and ensure that the child fulfils the criteria for conscious sedation. This technique usually requires an anaesthetist or similarly trained person to administer the nitrous oxide, as changes in level of consciousness demand alterations in concentrations of nitrous

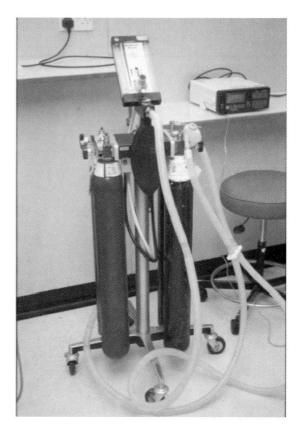

Fig. 2 A combined flow meter for nitrous oxide and oxygen and a mixture control allowing the delivery of a variable concentration of nitrous oxide (0–70%).

oxide that are delivered to the patient.[15] Although widely used for relative analgesia for adult dental patients, this form of sedation does not seem to have gained popularity in paediatric units in the UK.

EFFICACY OF NITROUS OXIDE IN PAINFUL PROCEDURES

Nitrous oxide has been used in a wide variety of painful procedures (Table 2). Although many of the procedures listed in Table 2 were completed using nitrous oxide alone, many centres successfully used a combination of simple analgesics, local anaesthetic agents, and psychological approaches with nitrous oxide.[16–19,26]

EFFICACY OF ENTONOX® AND OTHER 50:50 MIXES OF NITROUS OXIDE AND OXYGEN

To describe the efficacy of nitrous oxide it is necessary to look at the work published at each concentration of nitrous oxide separately. For simplicity we have combined the work published on Entonox® with that of other 50:50 mixtures of nitrous oxide and oxygen, as they are identical in composition and mode of presentation and differ only in the mode of delivery of the agent mixture.

A national prospective survey of the use of 50% nitrous oxide and 50% oxygen in France analysed 1019 inhalations by children in a 2-month period. An additional systemic drug was used in 17.9% of these inhalations (midazolam 63%, acetaminophen 18%, nalbuphine 8.5%, hydroxyzine 5%, flunitrazepam 2%, chlorazepate 2%, morphine 1%, lorazepam 0.5%). EMLA cream was applied in 98.6% of lumbar punctures, 93.7% of bone marrow aspirations and 54.2% of lymph node or renal biopsies and lignocaine was infiltrated in 51% of minor surgical procedures, 40% of laceration repairs and 28% of bone marrow aspirates. Overall, 93% of children able to answer would accept nitrous oxide analgesia for a new painful procedure, and 88% of the staff were either satisfied or very satisfied with the technique.[19]

The use of Entonox® and 50:50 nitrous oxide/oxygen mix during painful procedures on children has also been described by groups from Derbyshire Children's Hospital,[16] Sheffield Children's Hospital,[17] Great Ormond Street Hospital for Children[18] (all Entonox®) and Service de pediatre, Centre Hospitalier, Cornouaille, France[22] (50:50 mix). These institutions report experience in a wide range of procedures (see Table 2.) and have assessed analgesia as excellent or good in 93% of cases (Derbyshire),[16] 57% of cases (Sheffield),[17] and 83.4% of cases (Cornouaille).[22] Effective analgesia and sedation has also been reported in children when using nitrous oxide/oxygen 50:50 for gastrointestinal endoscopy[21] and percutaneous renal biopsy.[23] There are very few randomised studies comparing the effectiveness of a 50:50 mixture of nitrous oxide and oxygen in providing analgesia during painful procedures in children.

Brislin compared the response to venepuncture of midazolam premedicated children (8 years and older) who were randomised to one of three groups: (i) nitrous oxide + EMLA cream; (ii) nitrous oxide + intradermal lidocaine; and (iii) nitrous oxide alone. Analgesia was rated as equal and adequate in all groups and there were no differences in the degree of sedation. There was, however, a higher incidence of withdrawal and vocalisation with venepuncture in the nitrous oxide alone group.[26]

Gall reported a reduction in pain-related behaviour and pain ratings during venepuncture with both 50% nitrous oxide and EMLA cream. Although EMLA was responsible for a delay of 28 ± 5 min it was more effective than nitrous oxide in the 1–4 year age group.[24]

During fracture manipulation, Gregory reported no significant difference in the amount of pain experienced between two groups of children who had been randomised to receive either 50:50 nitrous oxide/oxygen or an intravenous regional anaesthesia with lidocaine. Completion of the procedure was significantly quicker in the nitrous oxide group.[20] A 50:50 nitrous oxide/oxygen mix was also compared with intramuscular meperidine (pethidine) and promethazine in two randomised groups during fracture manipulation. The nitrous oxide group reported 100% satisfaction with the technique (compared with 53% satisfaction in the intramuscular group) and spent, on average, only 30 min in the out-patient department (53 min less than the intramuscular group).[27]

A prospective, randomised, placebo-controlled, double-blind comparison of 50:50 nitrous oxide/oxygen mix with 100% oxygen during the repair of lacerations in children aged 2–7 years showed no significant difference in pain scores, but the nitrous oxide group showed significantly less anxiety.[25] Another prospective randomised trial looked at laceration repair in children aged 2–6 years. The children received standard care (comforting, topical and injected lidocaine) alone, standard care with 50:50 nitrous oxide/oxygen mix, standard care and oral midazolam or standard care with midazolam and 50:50 nitrous oxide/oxygen mix. Nitrous oxide was reported to reduce distress more effectively and with fewer adverse effects than midazolam and also led to quicker recovery times.[28]

EFFICACY OF NITROUS OXIDE AT OTHER CONCENTRATIONS

The published literature regarding the efficacy for the use of nitrous oxide at concentrations higher than 50% is limited. Vetter compared the efficacy of 70% nitrous oxide with EMLA cream for paediatric venous cannulation in a randomised trial.[29] Patients in the nitrous oxide group reported significantly lower pain scores than the EMLA group. In a randomised trial, Henderson *et al.* compared the effect of 50% nitrous oxide, 70% nitrous oxide, 100% oxygen and no gas on pain during venous cannulation.[30] Children receiving 50% and 70% nitrous oxide were more relaxed and exhibited very little pain. However, children receiving 70% nitrous oxide developed more side-effects namely excitement, dysphoria and restlessness.

In a prospective study, children requiring painful procedures were administered nitrous oxide at a variable concentration ranging from 50–70% via a relative analgesia machine. The results revealed that children over the age of 6 years benefited the most in terms of analgesia and 93% of the patients fulfilled the criteria for conscious sedation.[31]

ADVERSE EFFECTS OF NITROUS OXIDE

Nitrous oxide has been widely used as an analgesic and sedative for over 150 years. Although the majority of its adverse effects are minor and transient, a thorough knowledge of the possible sequelae to nitrous oxide inhalation is essential.

The French survey of 1019 inhalations of 50:50 nitrous oxide/oxygen mix during painful procedures in children noted minor side-effects in 37% of cases. These effects were euphoria (20.1%), change in visual or auditory perception (7%), dreams (5.7%), nausea and vomiting (3.7%), deep sedation (2.1%), paraesthesia (1.7%), dizziness (1.6%), restlessness (1.5%), and nightmares (1.2%), all of which were transient and had vanished within 5 min.[19]

Minor side-effects during the use of nitrous oxide for painful procedures in children were also reported in 0%,[20] 0.6%,[22] 5.5%,[16] 14%,[31] 33%[23] and 58%[25] of cases, all were transient and disappeared on discontinuation of the gas.

Enclosed gas spaces

Due to its low blood solubility, nitrous oxide diffuses across tissue membranes 15 times more rapidly than oxygen and 25 times more rapidly than nitrogen. Nitrous oxide will consequently move rapidly into any gas-filled space within the body leading to an increase in its volume. This can be important clinically in the presence of pneumothorax, bowel obstruction, intra-cerebral air, gas embolus, post-myringoplasty, and in decompression sickness. Nitrous oxide is, therefore, contra-indicated in a number of situations (Table 3).

Table 3 Contra-indications to nitrous oxide use Group I

Pneumothorax	Following air encephalography
Severe bullous emphysema	Myringoplasty
Air or gas embolism	Decompression sickness
Intestinal obstruction	Recent underwater dive

Hypoxia

There have been some highly publicised cases of hypoxia and death secondary to the accidental administration of 100% nitrous oxide from anaesthetic machines. The Royal College of Anaesthetists now recommends that nitrous oxide should not be administered from machines that lack an 'anti-hypoxic linkage' system. In addition, machines should be checked prior to use and an oxygen analyser used at the fresh gas outlet.

Nitrous oxide for procedural pain is administered from either an Entonox® cylinder or via a relative analgesia machine ensuring the patient is simultaneously inhaling 30–50% oxygen at all times. This ensures a well-oxygenated child at all times and limits hypoxia.

When nitrous oxide was inhaled in concentrations of 50–70% during painful procedures in children, hypoxia was not reported but 9% of patients developed desaturation ($SaO_2 < 95\%$).[31] After midazolam pre-medication of 0.5 mg/kg, nitrous oxide up to 60% did not result in oxygen saturations of less than 92%, but did cause deep sedation in 1 child.[32]

In adults, nitrous oxide at 30% has been shown to have no effect on laryngeal reflexes,[33] but at higher concentrations and when combined with opioids and benzodiazepines deep sedation, airway obstruction oxygen desaturation and apnoea are more common in children.[34]

Diffusion hypoxia is a theoretical phenomenon that can occur when nitrous oxide inhalation is ceased. Nitrous oxide's rapid diffusion across the alveolar membrane can theoretically displace oxygen, so causing hypoxia. It is recommended practice, therefore, to administer high-flow oxygen for 5 min after discontinuing nitrous oxide.

Nausea and vomiting

The incidence of nausea and vomiting has been reported variously to be 7.8%,[31] less than 5%,[34] and 3.7%[19] when nitrous oxide is used for painful procedures in children. This side-effect is generally transient and is terminated by discontinuation of the gas. Appropriate fasting prior to the procedure may reduce the risk of aspiration if vomiting occurs.

Bowel function is unaltered after colonoscopy and abdominal surgery in adults if nitrous oxide is used during the procedure.[35]

Dysphoria, excitement and euphoria

Despite psychological support prior to and during the procedure, some children report dreams (5.7%),[19] nightmares (1.2%),[19] dysphoria (2%),[31] and excitement (4.4%).[31] These again are transient and disappear on discontinuation of the gas.

Euphoria can occur as demonstrated by these comments from children who had received Entonox® in Derby: 'it made me tell the nurses I love them'; 'it made me feel fizzy'; and 'I was very giggly'.[16]

Vitamin synthesis

Nitrous oxide can inhibit the enzyme methionine synthase and interfere with folate metabolism, so impairing DNA synthesis. Prolonged exposure can, therefore, impair bone marrow function and lead to a condition identical to that seen with vitamin B_{12} deficiency.[36]

In clinical practice, nitrous oxide is very rarely used frequently enough by the same patient for bone marrow changes to occur. If nitrous oxide is administered more frequently than every 2–4 days and for more than 6–12 h, blood samples should be taken and examined for megaloblastic anaemia and leukopenia.[37] Chronic inhalation as seen in recreational use and abuse can lead to full-blown megaloblastic anaemia or subacute combined degeneration of the cord.

One adult patient was exposed to nitrous oxide daily over a 7-month period for dressing changes and prolonged orthopaedic operations. After his last exposure of 4 h, he developed megaloblastic anaemia, encephalopathy and classical subacute combined degeneration of the cord. All these abnormalities resolved on discontinuation of the nitrous oxide and vitamin B_{12} replacement.[38]

Occupational exposure and staff safety

There has been concern about the effects on staff of the long-term exposure to nitrous oxide. Animal models have shown that 24 h of exposure at levels of 1000 ppm, and shorter exposures at critical times of pregnancy to 50–70% can lead to an increased incidence of fetal resorptions and abnormalities.[36] These findings have not been repeated in human studies. A study of 4000 midwives showed that occupational exposure to nitrous oxide was not associated with an increased risk of abortion.[39]

The Health and Safety Committee has set an occupational exposure limit of 100 ppm over an 8 h period, this is a fifth of the dose at which no effects were seen in animal studies.[13]

To reduce environmental exposure, treatment areas should be well ventilated to maintain 7–10 air exchanges/hour. If possible, expired gases should be removed by a scavenging system.

Up to 20% of medical and dental students have used nitrous oxide 'socially'.[36] Recreational abuse of nitrous oxide is a potential problem for the health of the staff so steps should be taken to prevent unauthorised use. The cylinders should be kept in a designated place, a record of their contents kept and the breathing apparatus removed after each treatment episode and stored separately.

Environmental pollution

The principal source of atmospheric nitrous oxide is from the breakdown of fertilisers and natural compounds in the soil. In the US, medical nitrous oxide only accounts for 0.5% of that released into the atmosphere. As it reduces atmospheric heat radiation, nitrous oxide does play a minor part in the 'green house effect'.[7]

Setting up a service

A number of recent publications have described the introduction of and initial experiences using Entonox® for painful procedures in children.[11-13] BOC Medical Gases have also produced a training video and guidelines for Entonox® use in painful procedures.[40]

When setting up a nitrous oxide for painful procedures service, consideration should be given to staff training, procedure suitability, patient selection, patient preparation, safety, post-procedure care and audit. Input from a multidisciplinary team including a consultant anaesthetist with an interest in paediatric pain, a consultant paediatrician, an accident and emergency consultant, paediatric nurses, the pain control team, a pharmacist and a play therapist or psychologist is ideal.

Staff training

A member of staff should be trained in the administration of nitrous oxide and in the monitoring of the patient during the procedure. There should **always** be a separate member of staff to perform the procedure while the trained member of staff administers the nitrous oxide and monitors the patient.

An initial theoretical course followed by the observation of nitrous oxide being administered by experienced staff. A period of supervised administrations followed by feedback and questions then proceeds to 'solo' administration. All staff should be trained in basic paediatric life support and have immediate access to identified senior medical help. Staff should receive on-going training and feedback on the success and problems of the service.

Procedure suitability

Painful procedures that are suitable to be done with nitrous oxide should be short, minimally invasive, not interfere with the route of administration of nitrous oxide and not result in severe post-procedure pain. An extensive list of suitable procedures is given in Table 2.

Patient selection

A member of the medical staff should initially assess any patient undergoing a medical procedure. Nitrous oxide is contra-indicated in patients where there is an air or gas filled space (Table 3). It is also contra-indicated in the circumstances listed in Table 4.

If there is any history or suspicion of airway obstruction or compromise, the patient should be assessed by an anaesthetist before administration of any sedative medication including nitrous oxide.

For self-administration of nitrous oxide, the patient must be able to understand and carry out the instructions given by the staff – very young or neurologically impaired children as well as those with communication or behavioural difficulties may, therefore, not be suitable. It is possible to give instructions via an interpreter if needed.

Younger children may not benefit as much from the use of nitrous oxide as explained above. In a reported series from France, children 3 years or younger demonstrated more crying and were evaluated to have experienced more pain

Table 4 Contra-indications to nitrous oxide use Group II

Contra-indication	Rationale
Head injuries with impaired consciousness	Sedation may confound neurological observation
Maxillo-facial injuries	Use of the mask or mouthpiece may be difficult
Heavily sedated or intoxicated patients	Increased sedation may lead to improper use of the equipment, vomiting and aspiration

than children older than 3 years.[19] When nitrous oxide for painful procedures was given via the relative analgesia machine, the best results were seen in children older than 6 years. Children younger than 6 years demonstrated poor technique and high anxiety towards mask application.[31]

Patient preparation

The patient's medical or nursing staff may make a referral for nitrous oxide analgesia. Once the child has been assessed and deemed suitable, an explanation of the benefits and possible side-effects of the technique should be given to him/her (if appropriate) and parents or guardians. Any psychological techniques such as distraction and imagery should be explained.

Some institutions insist on nitrous oxide being prescribed on the 'as required' portion of the patient's drug chart. Any simple analgesics such as paracetamol and NSAIDs should be administered as directed by the medical team.

The patient should be fasted (including nasogastric or percutaneous endoscopic gastrostomy feeds) for 2 h prior to the procedure. If sedative premedication is given, a 4-h fasting time should be observed.

Prior to the procedure starting, the patient should practice inhaling the nitrous oxide for 3 min as this allows them to become comfortable with the technique and this helps to create a steady-state of analgesia.

Safety

All equipment should be well maintained, clean and checked before use. Scavenging equipment should be available if possible. The procedure room used should be 'child friendly', well lit, warm and well ventilated. Some procedures such as chest drain removal or dressing changes can be done at the child's bed space on the ward. Full resuscitation equipment including suction should be immediately available.

The most important safety measure is the continued presence of a trained member of staff who continually monitors the condition and response of the child. Pulse oximetry should be used unless the child is having burns dressings changed in a bath.

After each session, all equipment should be cleaned, any mouth pieces or filters used disposed of and the level of nitrous oxide checked and new cylinders ordered if needed.

Post-procedure care

Supplementary oxygen should be given for 5–10 min after stopping nitrous oxide. The patient should be monitored for 30 min to ensure all effects of the nitrous oxide have worn off. When first mobilised, care should be taken that there is no residual dizziness or disorientation. Patients can return home on the same day as nitrous oxide inhalation. They should meet the discharge criteria as used by the individual institution's day surgery unit.

Details of every nitrous oxide administration, its efficacy and any side-effects should be kept in the patient's notes. As with all medical interventions, an on-going audit of cases, results and adverse incidents should be performed. This will help to plan for future provision of the service, identify any problems and be used in education of staff.

Key points for clinical practice

- Desirable characteristics of the ideal agent for painful procedures include sedation and analgesia.

- Conscious sedation is a technique in which the use of a drug or drugs produces a state of depression of the central nervous system enabling the painful procedure to be carried out with minimal distress.

- To ensure safety, the technique should ensure verbal contact with the patient throughout the period of sedation.

- Nitrous oxide, an analgesic and sedative with rapid onset and offset of action, is an ideal agent for painful procedures. The efficacy of nitrous oxide is attributed to its properties, which produce a sense of euphoria and detached attitude toward pain and surroundings.

- One of the most favourable characteristic is the short recovery time (< 5 min) which is ideal for out-patient procedures.

- Nitrous oxide can be delivered with oxygen at a fixed concentration of 50% (Entonox®) via prefilled cylinders or at a variable concentration (0–70%).

- Prospective surveys and randomised trials have shown nitrous oxide to be effective in reducing pain and anxiety during venepuncture, bone marrow aspiration, lumbar puncture, dressing changes, removal of chest drain and some orthopaedic manipulations.

- The incidence of minor side-effects such nausea/vomiting dysphoria and excitement is 7%, 2% and 4%, respectively. These are transient and disappear on discontinuation of the gas.

- The incidence of adverse effects associated with the inhalation of nitrous oxide and oxygen is minimal. However, a thorough knowledge of the possible adverse effects and prevention is essential.

Key points for clinical practice (continued)

- The administrator who can be a physician or nurse specialist should have prior training in the principle of conscious sedation using nitrous oxide. This includes patient selection, working knowledge of equipment, and acquisition of skills in monitoring the child's state of consciousness while inhaling nitrous oxide. It would be useful to enlist the help of an anaesthetist (ideally with an interest in paediatric pain) in setting up the service and training.

- Addition of opioids, benzodiazepines and chloral hydrate has been shown to increase the incidence of oxygen desaturation. The concomitant use of other agents that also depress the central nervous system should be discouraged in this setting.

- Addition of simple analgesics and local anaesthetics should be encouraged as they reduce post-procedural pain.

- Failure to alleviate distress during the procedure could be attributed to poor technique of administration and the mask actually increasing the child's anxiety. Children over the age of 3 years should receive pre-procedural education in the correct use of the mask. Cognitive therapy in the form of imagery and distraction and positive incentive should also be an integral part of the technique.

- Administration of nitrous oxide for painful procedures in very young children may not be as effective compared with older children.

References

1. Anderson CTM, Zeltzer LK, Fanurik D. Procedural pain. In: Schecter NL, Berde CB, Yaster M. (eds) *Pain in Infants, Children, and Adolescents*. Baltimore, MD: Williams & Wilkins, 1992.
2. Intercollegiate Working Party chaired by The Royal College of Anaesthetists. *Implementing and Ensuring Safe Sedation Practice for Healthcare in Adults*. London: The Royal College of Anaesthetists 2001 <www.rcoa.ac.uk/directorate_B.asp?DOC_ID=154>.
3. Sievers T, Yee J, Foley M. Midazolam for conscious sedation during pediatric oncology procedures: safety and recovery parameters. *Pediatrics* 1991; **88**: 1172–1179.
4. Marx CM, Stein J, Tyler MK. Ketamine-midazolam versus meperidine-midazolam for painful procedures in pediatric oncology patients. *J Clin Oncol* 1997; **15**: 94–102.
5. Tobias JD, Phipps S, Smith B. Oral ketamine premedication to alleviate the distress of invasive procedures in pediatric oncology patients. *Pediatrics* 1992; **90**: 537-541
6. Rushman GB, Davies NJH, Atkinson RS. *A Short History of Anaesthesia*. Oxford: Butterworth-Heinemann, 1996.
7. British Oxygen Company, Entonox® Medical Gas Data Sheet G4042. Guildford: British Oxygen Company, 1995.

8. Chapman WP, Arrowhead JG, Beecher HK. The analgesic effects of low concentrations of nitrous oxide compared in man with morphine sulphate. *J Clin Invest* 1943; **22**: 871–875.

9. Dundee JW, Moore J. Alterations in response to somatic pain. An evaluation of a method of analgesimitry. *Br J Anaesth* 1960; **32**: 396.

10. Maze M, Fujinaga M. Recent advances in understanding the actions and toxicity of nitrous oxide. *Anaesthesia* 2000; **55**: 311–314.

11. De lima J, Hatch D, Torsney C. Nitrous oxide analgesia – a 'sting in the tail'. *Anaesthesia* 2000; **55**: 932–933.

12. Fujinaga M, Doone R, Davies MF, Maze M. Nitrous oxide lacks the antinociceptive effect on the tail flick test in new-born rats. *Anesth Analg* 2000; **91**: 6–10.

13. British Oxygen Company. *Entonox Controlled Pain Relief*. Guildford: British Oxygen Company, 2000.

14. Roberts G. Inhalation sedation (relative analgesia) with oxygen/nitrous oxide gas mixtures. *Dent Update* 1990; **17**: 139–142.

15. Katzen B, Edwards K. Nitrous oxide analgesia for interventionl radiological procedures. *AJR Am J Roentgenol* 1983; **140**: 145–148.

16. Vater M, Hessell D. Nitrous oxide and oxygen mixture (Entonox®), and acute procedural pain. *Paediatr Perinat Drug Ther* 2000; **4**: 35–43.

17. Pickup S, Pagdin J. Procedural pain: Entonox can help. *Paediatr Nurs* 2001; **12**: 33–36.

18. Bruce E, Franck L. Self-administered nitrous oxide (Entonox®) for the management of procedural pain. *Paediatr Nurs* 2000; **12**: 15–19.

19. Annequin D, Carbajal R, Chauvin P, Gall O, Tournaire B, Murat I. Fixed 50% nitrous oxide oxygen mixture for painful procedures: a French survey. *Pediatrics* 2000; **105**: E47.

20. Gregory P, Sullivan A. Nitrous oxide compared with intravenous regional anaesthesia in pediatric forearm fracture manipulation. *J Pediatr Orthop* 1996; **16**: 187–191.

21. Michaud L, Gottrand F, Ganga-Zandzou P *et al*. Nitrous oxide sedation in pediatric patients undergoing gastrointestinal endoscopy. *J Pediatr Gastroenterol Nutr* 1999; **28**: 310–314.

22. Vic P, Laguette D, Blondin G *et al*. Utilisation of an equimolar mixture of oxygen-nitrous oxide in a general pediatric ward. *Arch Pediatr* 1999; **6**: 844–848.

23. Pietrement C, Salomon R, Monceaux F, Petitjean C, Niaudet P. Analgesia with oxygen-nitrous oxide mixture during percutaneous renal biopsy in children. *Arch Pediatr* 2001; **8**: 145–149.

24. Gall O, Annequin D, Ravault N, Murat I. Relative effectiveness of lignocaine-prilocaine emulsion and nitrous oxide inhalation for routine preoperative laboratory testing. *Paediatr Anaesth* 1999; **9**: 305–310.

25. Burton J, Auble T, Fuchs S. Effectiveness of 50% nitrous oxide/50% oxygen during laceration repair in children. *Acad Emerg Med* 1998; **5**: 112–117.

26. Brislin R, Stayer S, Schwartz R, Pasquariello C. Analgesia for venepuncture in a paediatric surgery centre. *J Paediatr Child Health* 1995; **31**: 542–544.

27. Evans J, Buckley S, Alexander A, Gilpin A. Analgesia for the reduction of fractures in children: a comparison of nitrous oxide with intramuscular sedation. *J Pediatr Orthop* 1995; **15**: 73–77.

28. Luhmann JD, Kennedy RM, Porter FL, Miller JP, Jaffe DM. A randomized clinic trial of continuous flow nitrous oxide and midazolam for sedation of young children during laceration repair. *Ann Emerg Med* 2001; **37**: 20–27.

29. Vetter T. A comparison of EMLA cream versus nitrous oxide for pediatric venous cannulation. *J Clin Anesth* 1995; **7**: 486–490.

30. Henderson JM, Spence DG, Komocar L, Bonn G, Stenstrom RJ. Administration of nitrous oxide to pediatric patients provides analgesia for venous cannulation. *Anesthesiology* 1990; **72**: 269–271.

31. Kanagasundaram SA, Lanae LJ, Cavalleto BP, Keneally JP, Cooper MG. Efficacy and safety of nitrous oxide in alleviating pain and anxiety during painful procedures. *Arch Dis Child* 2001; **84**: 492–495.

32. Litman RS, Berkowitz RJ, Ward DS. Levels of consciousness and ventilatory parameters in young children during sedation with oral midazolam and nitrous oxide. *Arch Pediatr Adolesc Med* 1996; **150**: 671–675.

33. Roberts GJ, Wignall BK. Efficacy of the laryngeal reflex during oxygen-nitrous oxide sedation (relative analgesia). *Br J Anaesth* 1982; **54**: 1277–1281.
34. Gall O, Annequin D, Benoit G, Van Glabeke E, Vrancea F, Murat I. Adverse events of premixed nitrous oxide and oxygen for procedural sedation in children. *Lancet* 2001; **358**: 1514–1515.
35. Krogh B, Jorn JP, Henneberg SW. Nitrous oxide does not influence operating conditions or postoperative course in colonic surgery. *Br J Anaesth* 1994; **72**: 55–57.
36. Brodsky JB, Cohen EN. Adverse effects of nitrous oxide. *Med Toxicol* 1986; **1**: 362–374.
37. BOC Medical. *Entonox Protocol Template*. Guildford: BOC Medical Gases, 2000.
38. King M, Coulter C, Boyle RS, Whitby MR. Neurotoxicity from overuse of nitrous oxide. *Med J Aust* 1995; **163**: 50–51.
39. Ahlborg Jr G, Axelsson G, Bodin L. Shift work, nitrous oxide exposure and spontaneous abortion among Swedish midwives. *Occup Environ Med* 1996; **53**: 374–378.
40. BOC Medical, The Priestley Centre, The Surrey Research Park, Guildford, Surrey GU2 7XY, UK.

Kate Khair Ian M. Hann Ri Liesner

6

The investigation of easy bruising

Bruising and minor bleeding are common sequelae of the day-to-day rough and tumble of childhood. However, there are two distinct groups of children where bruising and/or bleeding is worse than one would expect given the clinical history; these are children with underlying bleeding disorders and those who are being non-accidentally injured. It is imperative that healthcare workers should be able to distinguish between these two groups of children in order to ensure that they come to no further harm, by initiating appropriate investigation and treatment. This chapter will address normal, easy and abnormal bruising, which investigations to undertake to establish a diagnosis, and give a brief description of the possible underlying bleeding disorders.

NORMAL BRUISING

Bruising is caused by the escape of blood from the vessels into the skin or subcutaneous tissue following injury – but what is 'normal' bruising? Carpenter[1] states that bruises in babies up to about 9 months of age are unusual as they are not usually independently mobile. He conducted a study into the prevalence of bruising in 175 babies (84 boys and 93 girls) aged 6–9 months seen in routine child development clinics in Northern England. Thirty-two bruises, all on the bony prominences of the lower limbs and head, were seen in 22 babies (12.4%). Seven babies had more than one bruise, caused by early mobilisation. This bruising is reported as normal with no concerns about child abuse.

Ms Kate Khair SRN RSCN MSc MCGI, Clinical Nurse Specialist in Haemophilia (for correspondence)
Professor Ian M. Hann MD MRCS FRCP FRCPCH FRCPath, Deputy Centre Director
Dr Ri Liesner MA MBBChir MD MRCP(Paed) MRCPath, Centre Director

The Haemophilia Comprehensive Care Centre, Great Ormond Street Hospital for Children NHS Trust, Great Ormond Street, London WC1N 3JH, UK
E-mail: khairk@gosh.nhs.uk

Sugar *et al.*[2] report that bruising is significantly more obvious in white children than in African/American children ($P < 0.007$) and that this is probably related to skin pigmentation and not less bruising. This should be borne in mind when investigating non-white children for bleeding disorders or non-accidental injury. The severity and frequency of bruising can alter with seasonal changes – more bruising is seen and reported in the summer months when children are more likely to be seen with abrasions and bruises following injury, when playing outside in light-weight clothing.[3]

The size and colour of bruises are often used in an attempt to age injury, to establish multiple injury over time and to exonerate adult carers in non-accidental injury cases. The colour of bruising changes from red to yellow/green as extra-cellular haemoglobin is broken down. However, there is no consensus to the timing of this – ranging from days to weeks depending on size of bruise, depth below the skin, severity of the force, connective tissue support at the site of injury (different sequence where there is loose skin, *e.g.* around the eye and genitalia), age and sex of child, skin pigmentation, and medication(s) being taken (*e.g.* steroids).[4] Thus, it is unlikely that any single bruise can be aged unless the specific injury can be recalled.

EASY BRUISING

There is wide inter-individual variation in the degree to which a child will bruise following a defined episode of trauma. This can make the distinction of 'normal' easy bruising and 'abnormal' easy bruising difficult for the clinician. It is important to consider the pattern and severity of bruising, drug and family history, and associated symptoms.[5] Toddlers will develop bruises following trauma to the head and lower limbs whilst in older children the 'normal' bruises that can be expected are usually on lower limb prominences. Unusual patterns of bruising or the presence of petechiae, purpura or significant recurrent mucosal bleeding should lead to the suspicion of an underlying bleeding disorder or non-accidental injury. Recent attempts have been made to score bruising in children who are known to have been physically abused and compare them to those who have not been abused to differentiate patterns of bruising. Although this may have some use, it cannot replace the complex qualitative analysis required in the majority of cases of child abuse.[6]

All cases should have a detailed family history taken, including consanguinity, neonatal death, menorrhagia or post-partum haemorrhage, post-surgical (including religious circumcision) and dental bleeding going back several generations. In the drug history, all medications should be recorded including readily available over-the-counter medications used to treat fever. Even a single dose of non-steroidal anti-inflammatory drugs, which are frequently used by parents to treat febrile illness, can predispose to easy bruising which may persist for weeks or months.[7] There are a number of other regularly used drugs, such as those for anti-epileptic therapy, which can predispose to easy bruising as they can also affect platelet function (Table 1).

ABNORMAL BRUISING – IS IT NON-ACCIDENTAL INJURY?

When a child presents with significant bruising and/or bleeding, the health-care worker is faced with a dilemma as to whether the child has been a subject

Table 1 Drugs which may affect platelet function

Cytotoxic therapy	Diazepam
Ethanol	Sodium valproate
Chloramphenicol	Carbemazepine
Arsenic	Frusemide
Benzene	Tolbutamide
Non-steroidal anti-inflammatory drugs	Digoxin
Aspirin	Heparin
Rifampicin	Warfarin
Penicillin	Methyldopa
Sulphonamides	Oxyprenolol
Trimethoprim	Quinine

of non-accidental injury (NAI) or has a previously undiagnosed haemostatic disorder[8] – or, indeed, whether a child with a bleeding disorder has also been non-accidentally injured.[9–11] It is important to remember that NAI is probably more common than bleeding disorders, but that they are not mutually exclusive problems.[10,11] In every case, all options should be considered. NAI can present in many forms, including neglect, psychological, sexual, and physical abuse. It may present with: (i) bruising which may be abnormal in relation to both the site of the bruise and its severity out of proportion to the history; or (ii) more severe bleeding manifestations, such as intracranial bleeding,[12] and/or retinal haemorrhage.[13,14] Retinal haemorrhages are an uncommon finding in children with known bleeding disorders[15] and they have rarely been seen at diagnosis in children with leukaemia.[16] Intracranial bleeding, however, is occasionally seen in children with bleeding disorders, usually following birth injury or head trauma.[17] A further issue that may cause confusion is that previously haemostatically normal children have been reported to develop coagulation defects, such as isolated prolonged prothrombin times or disseminated intravascular coagulation following traumatic brain injury.[12,18] Bony fractures in association with haemorrhage are common in suspected cases of NAI and a positive skeletal survey makes an underlying haemostatic defect less likely because there are no known associations of bony fragility and coagulation defects. In those cases in which a coagulation factor or platelet defect is at all possible, it is essential that these children be screened for the rare, as well as common, bleeding disorders. Initial screening investigations are listed in Table 2 and, if all normal, these exclude *only* the commonest conditions which cause serious bleeding following trauma or spontaneous bleeding. They do not exclude a number of other important conditions that need to be excluded (Table 3). Rare disorders such as Glanzmann's thrombasthenia or factor XIII deficiency[8,17] can present with intracranial haemorrhage and common, mild disorders such as type 1 von Willebrand's disease or mild platelet function defects can result in more serious bleeding than usually seen following traumatic episodes.[19] None of these conditions affect either the full blood count or the coagulation screen in many cases.

Table 2 Investigation of a suspected bleeding disorder – initial investigations

- History including detailed family and drug history
- Physical examination
- Full blood count and film
- Coagulation screen – PT, APTT, TT
- If PT or APTT prolonged do 50:50 mix with normal plasma to distinguish between possible factor deficiency or presence of inhibitor
- Fibrinogen, D-dimers
- Biochemical screen including renal and hepatic function tests

PT, prothrombin time; APTT, activated partial thromboplastin time; TT, thrombin time.

The complexity of many of the cases of abnormal bruising/bleeding or suspected NAI means that consultation with, or referral to, a paediatric haematology department for further assessment may be required. In the majority of cases and particularly in those in which there are no fractures, interpretation of screening test results as normal and equating this to normal haemostasis in an individual child is potentially medically negligent.[12] We would recommend that the case reports of all children with a potential diagnosis of NAI should be discussed with a paediatric haematologist and, where necessary, thorough investigation of the haemostatic system should be undertaken.

If the abnormal bruising is not a result of a haemostatic disorder or non-accidental injury the clinician must consider rare diseases such as collagen disorders and malignancy.[20,21] Collagen disorders (*e.g.* Ehlers-Danlos or Marfan's syndrome) have an increased bruising tendency because vascular integrity, which may be defective in these disorders, is essential for effective primary haemostasis. Capillary and skin elasticity is compromised and predisposes to bruising[22] and/or scarring. In some children, a simple test of thumb hyper-flexibility is sufficient to identify these conditions,[23] but this is not the case in all and may require expert advice from a rheumatologist or geneticist.

Table 3 Haemostatic disorders which may present with normal full blood count and normal coagulation screen

- Mild von Willebrand's disease
- Mild haemophilia A or B
- Mild factor XI deficiency
- Factor XIII deficiency
- α_2-Antiplasmin deficiency
- Plasminogen activator inhibitor-1 deficiency
- Glanzmann's thrombasthenia
- Platelet storage pool disease
- Platelet release defect
- Collagen disorders

Causes of bruising and bleeding in children and suggested guidelines for investigation are described in the following sections.

INITIAL INVESTIGATIONS

The initial investigations that are required in any case where a bleeding disorder or NAI is suspected are outlined in Table 2. These should be performed in the district general hospital laboratory. The results of these first-line tests may help to make a preliminary diagnosis as to whether the bruising is due to a platelet disorder, coagulation defect or potentially to NAI, but great care must be taken to remember that the conditions listed in Table 3 may not be detected by the baseline investigations in Table 2.

PLATELET DISORDERS – THROMBOCYTOPAENIA

The full blood count in the initial screen will indicate if there is a quantitative platelet abnormality. Thrombocytopaenia can be either an isolated finding or part of a generalized bone marrow failure condition and, like qualitative disorders, can be congenital (rare) or acquired (common). The platelet count should be repeated to ensure that the first count is not artefactually lowered by platelet clumping or clotting of the sample. Once thrombocytopaenia has been confirmed, the conditions that should be considered are listed in Table 4.

By far the commonest cause of thrombocytopaenia in childhood is immune thrombocytopaenic purpura (ITP), which is usually an acquired self-limiting post-viral condition.[7] The autoantibody produced is usually IgG directed against antigens on the platelet membrane. Antibody-coated platelets are removed by the reticulo-endothelial system, reducing the life-span of the platelet to a few hours. The platelet count can vary from $< 5 \times 10^9/l$ to near normal. The severity of bleeding is less than that seen with comparable degrees of thrombocytopaenia in bone marrow failure due to the predominance of young, larger and functionally superior platelets. Severe bleeding manifestations are rare when the platelet count is above $20 \times 10^9/l$.[24] A bone marrow aspirate, if performed, may show increased numbers of megakaryocytes and it may be possible to demonstrate antibody bound to the platelet surface by flow cytometry. If the thrombocytopaenia persists beyond a few weeks, referral to a paediatric haematologist should be considered, aiming to exclude a congenital platelet disorder (see below). Other causes of acquired thrombocytopaenia can also be antibody-mediated causing increased consumption of platelets such as in viral infections (*e.g.* HIV and EBV) or the cause can be a micro-angiopathic process such as in haemolytic uraemic syndrome and disseminated intravascular coagulation.[25] A low platelet count is a common presenting feature of bone marrow malignancies such as acute leukaemias,[26] myelodysplasia,[27] or a bone marrow failure disorder such as aplastic anaemia.[28] There are often other abnormalities in the blood count, such as neutropaenia or anaemia, which suggest that a bone marrow examination is required for diagnosis.

Congenital thrombocytopaenias are rare, but may manifest either soon after birth or in toddler-hood when mobility increases and when personal accidents are most common. Thrombocytopaenia with absent radii ('TAR syndrome') is an autosomal recessive disorder characterized by bilateral absence of the radii,

Table 4 Congenital and acquired platelet disorders

Congenital platelet disorders

- *Thrombocytopaenias*
    - Amegakaryocytic thrombocytopaenia
    - Thrombocytopaenia with absent radii – TAR syndrome
    - Wiskott-Aldrich syndrome
    - May Hegglin anomaly
    - Fanconi's anaemia
    - Bernard Soulier syndrome (with platelet dysfunction)
    - Gray platelet syndrome (with platelet dysfunction)

- *Platelet dysfunction*
    - Glanzmann's thrombasthenia
    - Platelet storage pool disease
        - Idiopathic
        - Hermansky-Pudlak syndrome
    - Chediak Higashi syndrome
    - Platelet release defects
    - Platelet-type von Willebrand's disease

Acquired platelet disorders

- *Thrombocytopaenia due to bone marrow failure/replacement*
    - Drug-induced including cytotoxic therapy
    - Malignancies – leukaemia, metastatic tumour, myelodysplasia
    - Aplastic anaemia
    - Associated with infection

- *Thrombocytopaenia due to increased consumption of platelets*
    - Autoimmune – idiopathic thrombocytopaenic purpura
    - Infection-associated – infectious mononucleosis, HIV, malaria
    - Drug-induced – heparin, paenicillin, *etc.*
    - Haemolytic uraemic syndrome/thrombotic thrombocytopaenic purpura
    - Hypersplenism and splenomegaly
    - Disseminated intravascular coagulation
    - Massive transfusion syndrome

- *Acquired platelet dysfunction*
    - Aspirin and non-steroidal anti-inflammatory agents
    - Anti-epileptic therapy
    - Penicillins and cephalosporins
    - Uraemia
    - Liver disease
    - Cardiopulmonary bypass
    - Fish oils

which is clinically obvious at birth. The thrombocytopaenia in this disorder improves over time with most children having normal platelet counts at 7 or 8 years of age.[29] This must be differentiated from amegakaryocytic thrombocytopaenia, which (like Fanconi's anaemia)[30] is a pre-leukaemic condition. Wiskott-Aldrich syndrome[31] is an X-linked immune deficiency disorder associated with eczema and small platelets in which children are prone to bacterial infections, which may be frequent and severe. Bruising is most commonly seen within the first 6 months of life and may precede the onset of recurrent infections. Gray platelet syndrome[32] is due to platelet alpha granule deficiency and results in severe bruising and bleeding from an early age. There is mild thrombocytopaenia and abnormal platelet function causing defective platelet aggregation. Examination of the blood film by light or electron microscopy usually makes the diagnosis as agranular platelets are seen. Bernard-Soulier syndrome[33] is also an important cause of a severe bruising/bleeding tendency from infancy. It is an autosomal recessive disorder most commonly seen in consanguineous families. It presents with moderate thrombocytopaenia (30–80 x 10^9/l), giant platelets, bruising and mucous membrane bleeding. In this condition, the platelets fail to aggregate with ristocetin due to the characteristic absence of glycoprotein 1b on the platelet surface. The May Hegglin anomaly is a rare autosomal dominant condition causing mild thrombocytopaenia, giant platelets and a bleeding tendency, which is usually trivial.[34]

PLATELET FUNCTION (QUALITATIVE) DISORDERS

Transient abnormalities in platelet function causing temporary bruising are common following ingestion of non-steroidal anti-inflammatory drugs or aspirin, which is sometimes used therapeutically as an anti-platelet agent in paediatric practice. Acquired platelet dysfunction is also a common complication of uraemia or liver disease and can also follow cardio-pulmonary bypass procedures.[32]

Inherited platelet function defects are rare but may result in profound, life-long bruising and/or bleeding. The most severe of these is Glanzmann's thrombasthenia,[32,33] a rare autosomal recessive disorder in which the platelets are normal in number and size, but have decreased or absent expression of the membrane glycoprotein IIb/IIIa which is crucial for effective platelet aggregation and clot propagation *in vivo*. It presents early in life, frequently in infancy, with severe, often spontaneous bleeding usually from the mucous membranes, which can be life threatening if there is a delay in treatment. Petechiae are common (especially following restriction for venesection) and bruising is usually extensive following even trivial injury. Platelet storage pool disorders with a deficiency in the nucleotide content of the dense granules of the platelet can be idiopathic or part of a more complex disorder.[7,32] Generally, they cause a mild-to-moderate bruising tendency, but in some children there is brisk bleeding following trauma or surgery. Inheritance is poorly understood, though it is known that Wiskott Aldrich syndrome, which can be associated with a storage pool disorder, is X-linked and Hermansky Pudlack[35] syndrome is autosomal recessive. The latter is a disorder characterized by oculocutaneous albinism and storage pool disorder. The bleeding tendency is usually mild, but there are case reports in the literature that demonstrate how, on rare occasions, spontaneous bleeding may occur.[19] Albinism is also a feature of Chediak Higashi syndrome in which there are characteristic giant organelles in leukocytes, susceptibility to infection and mental retardation.[34] Platelet release defects also cause a mild bruising/bleeding tendency. This is a heterogeneous group of disorders of signal transduction or thromboxane generation resulting in poor granule release on platelet activation.[24,32]

INVESTIGATION OF A SUSPECTED PLATELET DISORDER

Figure 1 is a flow chart with a proposed scheme of investigation for easy bruising and includes appropriate tests for a suspected platelet disorder. Table 5 shows the

Table 5 Interpretation of laboratory tests in platelet defects

Disorder/syndrome	Inheritance	Platelet number	Platelet size	Aggregation				Confirmatory tests
				ADP	Coll	Arach	Rist	
Glanzmann's thrombasthenia	AR	N	N	0	0	0	N	GP IIb/IIIa ↓ on flow
Bernard-Soulier	AR	↓	↑	N	N	N	0	GP Ib/IX ↓ on flow
Storage pool disease	AD/AR	N	N	→	→	→	N	ADP ATP content/release ↓
Hermansky Pudlak	AR	N	N	→	→	V	N	ADP ATP content/release ↓
Wiskott-Aldrich syndrome (WAS) content/release ↓	XLR	→	→	→	→	→	N	WAS gene studies; ADP ATP
Chediak Higashi	AR	V	N	→	→	V	N	ADP ATP content/release ↓
May Hegglin	AD	→	↑	N	N	N	N	Film/family testing
Gray platelet	AR	V	↑	V	V	V	N	Film/EM/Flow for α-granule marker
Platelet release	V	N	N	N	N	0	N	ADP ATP release ↓
ITP	–	↓↓	V	*	*	*	*	Bone marrow; autoimmune screen

AR, autosomal recessive; AD, autosomal dominant; ADP, adenosine diphosphate; ATP, adenosine triphosphate; Coll, collagen; Arach, arachidonic acid; Rist, ristocetin; XLR, X-linked recessive; 0, no aggregation/agglutination; V, variable; N, normal; ↓, decreased; ↑, increased; GP, glycoprotein; EM, electron microscopy; *not usually possible due to very low platelet count.

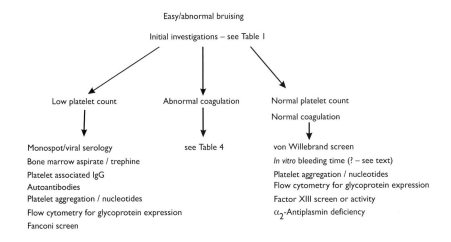

Fig. 1 Suggested scheme for investigation of easy bruising (note not all investigations will be required for all patients).

characteristic findings in many of the conditions described above. Unfortunately, if a platelet disorder is suspected, the gold-standard investigation remains platelet aggregation and measurement of platelet nucleotides, which are only performed in large, well-equipped laboratories and require a minimum of 20 ml blood. There is no reliable screening test available to date; the template bleeding time is no longer performed as it is invasive and unreliable. Even though there are now *in vitro* bleeding time devices available which will detect the severe disorders, such as Glanzmann's thrombasthenia and Bernard Soulier syndrome, they are unreliable with milder platelet disorders which may well contribute to the severity of bruising in a small child. However, the one situation in which the PFA-100® *in vitro* device has an important role is in infants who present with bleeding or bruising where the cause is unclear. A small volume of blood aspirated into this machine will reliably tell the clinician whether severe disorders such as Glanzmann's thrombasthenia or Bernard-Soulier syndrome are a possible diagnosis.[36]

COAGULATION DISORDERS

If initial investigations suggest that a coagulation disorder may be the cause of bruising, further investigations are required. Interpretation of an abnormality in the initial coagulation screen and further tests required are detailed in Table 6, although not all haematology laboratories will have all these in their repertoire of available tests. The majority of children with persistent abnormalities of coagulation screening will have an underlying bleeding disorder[37] and, therefore, such cases should be discussed with, and referred to, a paediatric haematologist and/or a haemophilia comprehensive care centre. Inherited coagulation disorders and congenital platelet disorders are relatively rare; current national guidelines recommend that all children are cared for by multidisciplinary teams with expertise in this area. The classification of the most important coagulation disorders in children is shown in Table 7, and the

Table 6 Interpretation and further investigation of coagulation screen results

PT	APTT	TT	Possible abnormality/Further investigation required
↑	N	N	• Factor VII deficiency (extrinsic pathway) • Liver disease • Vitamin K deficiency *Measurement of PT-based factors*
N	↑	N	• Deficiency of factor VIII (due to haemophilia or vWD) factors IX, XI, XII or contact factors (intrinsic pathway) *Measurement of APTT-based factors and von Willebrand screen – VIIIc, vWRAg, functional vW assay, e.g. vW Ricof or vW CBA* • Lupus anticoagulant or other coagulation factor inhibitor (prolongation does not correct with normal plasma) *DRVVT, Exner, KCT ACL*
N	N	↑	• Hypofibrinogenaemia • Dysfibrinogenaemia *Reptilase time and other thrombin time corrections*
↑	↑	N	• Deficiency of factors II, V, X (common pathway) • Vitamin K deficiency • Liver disease • Massive transfusion • Oral anticoagulants *PT- and APTT-based factors, INR*
N	↑	↑	• Heparin *Reptilase time and other thrombin time corrections*
↑	↑	↑	• Disseminated intravascular coagulation • Large amounts heparin • Severe hypofibrinogenaemia *D-dimers, reptilase time and other thrombin time corrections*
N	N	N	• All tests normal but history of bleeding – consider: • Mild vWD or haemophilia • Factor XIII deficiency • α_2-Antiplasmin deficiency • Platelet disorder (see Tables 2 & 3) *von Willebrand screen, factor XIII screen (clot stability test) or factor XIII activity α_2-antiplasmin level*

PT, prothrombin time; APTT, activated partial thromboplastin time; TT, thrombin time; N, within normal range, ↑, prolonged; vWD, von Willebrand's disease; VIIIc, factor VIII coagulant activity; vWRAg, von Willebrand factor related antigen; vW Ricof, von Willebrand factor ristocetin co-factor activity; vW CBA, collagen binding assay, DRVVT, dilute Russell viper venom time; KCT, kaolin cephalin time; ACL, anticardiolipin antibodies; INR, international ratio.

most important clinical and laboratory features of haemophilia and von Willebrand's disease are described in Table 8.

Haemophilia is an X-linked condition in which boys experience bruising and bleeding that can be severe.[37] Haemophilia A or classical haemophilia is a deficiency of factor VIII coagulant activity (FVIIIc) and affects about 1 in 10,000 boys. Haemophilia B or Christmas disease is a deficiency of factor IX and

Table 7 Coagulation disorders in children – classification

Inherited
- Haemophilia A
- Haemophilia B
- von Willebrand's disease
- Deficiency of factors II, V, VII, X, XI, XII or XIII
- Dys- or hypofibrinogenaemia
- α_2-Antiplasmin deficiency

Acquired
- Vitamin K deficiency
- Liver disease
- Disseminated intravascular coagulation
- Massive transfusion syndrome
- Dys- or hypofibrinogenaemia
- Disorders associated with malignancy
- Coagulation inhibitors

affects about 1 in 50,000 boys. The bruising/bleeding tendency correlates well with the plasma level of factor VIII/IX and 'runs true' in families. Approximately one-third of all boys diagnosed with haemophilia have no previous family history and have a new genetic mutation in their factor VIII or factor IX gene. It is typical for boys with severe haemophilia (factor VIII or factor IX level < 0.01 IU/ml; normal = 0.5–1.5 IU/ml) to present with severe bruising and joint bleeds between 6–12 months of age. Those with mild or moderate haemophilia (factor level > 0.02 IU/ml) may present later in childhood with trauma-related bruising or excessive bleeding following surgery or dental extraction. Carrier females of haemophilia may also suffer from mild bruising as they often have factor levels below the lower limit of normal.

von Willebrand's disease is the commonest inherited bleeding disorder with an incidence that is estimated at 1 in 100–1000.[37–39] It affects boys and girls equally, and inheritance is autosomal dominant or recessive depending on the sub-type, though there is variable penetrance. It is a very common cause of excess bruising and, therefore, any child with bruising that is not normal should be investigated for this disorder. The bruising is caused by quantitative or qualitative defect in von Willebrand factor, which is important for platelet adhesion in primary haemostasis. There are three major sub types of von Willebrand's disease: bleeding in type 1 and 2 is usually mild/moderate, but in type 3, where there is an absence of factor VIII and von Willebrand factor, the bruising/bleeding is usually severe especially from mucous membranes. In type 2B, there is associated thrombo-cytopaenia with enhanced sensitivity to ristocetin on platelet aggregometry. The diagnosis of the mildest and commonest form of von Willebrand's disease (type 1) can be difficult and may require blood samples on at least 3 occasions as these children can have levels of factor VIII and von Willebrand factor that are just above or just below the lower limit of the normal range and, as both these proteins are 'acute phase reactants', the levels can be raised by stress or infections, *etc*. The situation is further complicated as children who are blood group O have

Table 8 Clinical and laboratory features of haemophilia and von Willebrand's disease

	Haemophilia A or B	von Willebrand's disease
Inheritance	X-linked	Autosomal dominant (type 1 & 2) Autosomal recessive (type 3)
Molecular defect	**A**: Deletions or point mutations in factor VIII gene – Xq2.8 **B**: Deletions or point mutations in factor IX gene – Xq2.6	**Type 1**: Underlying genetic defects still under evaluation **Types 2 & 3**: Deletions or mutations involving different parts of large vWF gene – 12p2.1
Classification	**Mild**: FVIII/IX 0.05–0.5 IU/ml **Moderate**: 0.01–0.05 IU/ml **Severe**: <0.01 IU/ml	**Type 1**: Levels of FVIII and vWF mildly reduced (> 75% of cases) **Type 2**: Qualitative defects in vWF (20% of cases) **Type 3**: Levels of FVIII & vWF reduced to < 0.05 IU/ml (< 5% of cases)
Type of bleeding	**Mild**: Post-traumatic/post-surgical bleeding **Moderate**: As in mild with occasional spontaneous bleeds **Severe**: Frequent, severe muscle and joint bleeds	**Type 1**: Post-traumatic/post-surgical bleeding, easy bruising **Type 2**: As in type 1 with more mucosal, skin bleeding, epistaxis **Type 3**: Frequent, severe mucosal bleeds. May have haemarthroses
PT/TT/platelet count	Normal	Normal (platelet count may be reduced in type 2B)
APTT	Prolonged	Prolonged (may be at the upper end of normal range in type 1)
In vitro bleeding time	Normal	Increased (usually)
FVIIIc level	Reduced in haemophilia A Normal in haemophilia B	Reduced (may be at lower end of normal range in type 2B)
FIX level	Normal in haemophilia A Reduced in haemophilia B	Normal
vWF level	Normal	Reduced (may be at lower end of normal range in type 2B)
Ristocetin-induced platelet aggregation	Normal	Impaired (platelets show enhanced sensitivity to ristocetin in type 2B)

vWF, von Willebrand factor.

physiologically lower levels of factor VIII and von Willebrand factor than those of other blood groups (> 0.37 IU/ml rather than > 0.5 IU/ml), though there is undoubtedly an overlap in that some blood group O subjects have levels between 0.37–0.5 IU/ml and are normal whilst some have type 1 von Willebrand's disease. Due to the complexity of establishing this diagnosis, UK recommendations are that the care of these children is also overseen by haemophilia comprehensive care centres, which will also facilitate the correct treatment approach if/when treatment is required.[37–39]

Other coagulation factor deficiencies are rare compared to the conditions described above, but severe forms of some of them can result in a profound, life-threatening bleeding diathesis and making the correct diagnosis early is paramount to avoid death from bleeding or significant morbidity. Clinical features of these disorders are described briefly below.

Factors II, V, VII, and X deficiencies[8,40–42] cause significant bleeding when inherited as a homozygous characteristic, but heterozygotes can also have a mild bleeding/bruising tendency. The severe phenotypes may present in the neonatal period with severe bleeding and intracerebral haemorrhage; such infants are commonly born of consanguineous parents. Plasma levels of the deficient factor do not necessarily correlate with degree of bleeding diathesis.

Factor XI deficiency is inherited as an autosomal recessive trait – most commonly seen in Ashkenazi Jews. The bleeding tendency is usually mild in both homozygotes and heterozygotes, and the plasma level of circulating factor XI does not correlate well with bleeding tendency.[8,43]

Factor XII deficiency is commonly seen but rarely, if ever, predisposes to bruising/bleeding; therefore, it does not require correction prior to surgery.

Factor XIII deficiency is inherited as an autosomal recessive trait and homozygous inheritance results in factor XIII activity of < 0.05 IU/ml and a severe bleeding disorder as activated factor XIII stabilizes fibrin clots. This disorder commonly presents with umbilical cord bleeding and delay in cord separation or intracranial haemorrhage in the neonatal period. Bleeding is characteristically delayed for hours or days after the traumatic insult, and there is a healing defect with prominent scarring.[17]

Disorders of fibrinogen can be quantitative (hypo-/afibrinogenaemia) and/or qualitative (dysfibrinogenaemia). Hypofibrinogenaemia is probably the heterozygote form of homozygous afibrinogenaemia, which is a severe bleeding disorder usually presenting in early childhood.[40,44] Dysfibrinogenaemia may cause bleeding or thrombosis.[44]

α_2-Antiplasmin deficiency is an extremely rare abnormality of coagulation (13 cases reported in the literature) which does not affect clotting times *in vitro*. Thus, an α_2-antiplasmin level should be performed in children with a real bleeding diathesis and negative coagulation screens.[45] Another very rare defect that has been recognized to cause life-long bleeding is plasminogen activator inhibitor-1 deficiency which causes hyperfibrinolysis in affected patients.[46]

The development of an acquired disorder of coagulation in a child who is unwell from systemic or organ disease is generally much more common than congenital coagulation disorders. Vitamin K deficiency is probably the most common acquired bleeding disorder of childhood.[25,37,47] Vitamin K is required to synthesise factors II, VII, IX and X; deficiency can result in any degree of bleeding from minor bruising through to severe life-threatening haemorrhage. It is most commonly caused by conditions which cause liver dysfunction, gastrointestinal disorders and drug therapy particularly antibiotics and oral anticoagulants. In neonates and young infants, vitamin K deficiency can cause haemorrhagic disease of the new-born.[47] Neonates have low levels of vitamin K dependent factors at birth, there is absent gut synthesis of vitamin K, the liver is relatively immature, and there are low quantities of vitamin K in breast milk. Bleeding in haemorrhagic disease of the new-born can vary from bruising or petechiae in the first few days of life through to severe and life-threatening intracranial haemorrhage and/or gastrointestinal bleeding. Haemorrhagic disease of the new-born can be prevented by administration of i.m. vitamin K at birth.

Children with severe liver disease commonly have a coagulation disorder caused by: (i) impaired synthesis of coagulation factors; (ii) clearance of activated clotting factors; and (iii) enhanced fibrinolysis. There can also be an acquired platelet function defect. However, the liver has large reserves, so often only 10–15% of children have significant bleeding.[25]

Disseminated intravascular coagulation results from uncontrolled activation of the coagulation mechanism, causing unrestrained coagulation factor and platelet consumption, intravascular fibrin deposition, and accelerated degradation of fibrin and fibrinogen.[25]. It usually occurs in children who are critically ill and is best managed in an intensive care setting. The full list of causes can be found in any full paediatric or haematology text, but can be broadly categorised into severe infections, tissue or vascular injury or intravascular haemolysis (ABO incompatible transfusion, liver disease and malignancy). It can cause profuse bleeding into the skin, gastrointestinal tract and central nervous system. The laboratory findings include abnormalities in the coagulation screen (see Table 6) micro-angiopathic haemolysis as well as thrombocytopaenia, a low fibrinogen and elevated D-dimers.

Massive transfusion syndrome as a cause of coagulopathy is an unusual cause of bruising in paediatric practice, but occasionally a child will require a transfusion of blood equal to its blood volume within the period of a few hours. To avoid inappropriate use of blood products, the platelet count, coagulation screen and fibrinogen concentration should be monitored regularly.

Acquired dys- or hypofibrinogenaemia can occur in some systemic diseases in childhood, including renal or liver disease and following drug therapy, for example L-asparaginase and sodium valproate.[48]

Children with haematological abnormalities and malignancy usually present with low platelet counts suggesting bone marrow involvement. Occasionally, coagulation disorders occur such as disseminated intravascular coagulation, acquired factor deficiencies or von Willebrand's disease. The latter two conditions will present in a similar way to congenital abnormalities, but without a previous history or family history. These children should be referred to a specialist haemato-oncology centre for treatment with co-existent haemostasis expertise.

Coagulation inhibitors are rare in children who do not have an underlying inherited coagulation disorder.[49] They can occur in association with malignancy (see above) or occasionally post-surgery. Inhibitors to phospholipid (lupus anticoagulant) are more common, but are rarely associated with an excess bleeding risk except when the anti-phospholipid antibody is directed against prothrombin (factor II) and results in consumption of factor II. These usually follow viral infections and are generally transient.

Key points for clinical practice

- Bruising on bony prominences is the normal sequelae of childhood trauma. Bruising in other areas with or without a history of trauma may indicate that a child has an underlying bleeding disorder or that they are being non-accidentally injured.

- Non-accidental injury and bleeding disorders are not mutually exclusive and children with bleeding disorders are not immune to non-accidental injury.

- Laboratory investigation of easy bruising should include a full blood count and blood film, a coagulation screen (including PT, PTT, TT, fibrinogen and D-dimers and 50:50 mix if any of these are prolonged), renal and hepatic function tests. These alone, may establish a diagnosis.

- If an abnormality in the full blood count or coagulation screen is identified, further investigation and/or treatment at a specialist centre should be considered.

- Frequently used over-the-counter medicines, e.g. Ibuprofen (Junifen or Nurofen) or aspirin-containing drugs, may predispose to easy bruising as they affect platelet function as do some commonly used antibiotics.

- A comprehensive family and drug history will inform the haematology team of potential diagnoses.

- Bruising may be the first clinical sign of systemic diseases such as HIV, leukaemia, bone marrow failure or liver disease.

- Inherited bleeding disorders are relatively rare, but many are autosomal recessive and a new causative mutation can arise. Therefore, the child in question may be the first family member to be clinically affected.

- Children with bleeding disorders should be treated at recognised paediatric centres, where paediatric haematologists, nurses and professionals allied to medicine will ensure appropriate treatment, genetic analysis and counselling for family members.

- In children with normal screening tests, where there is evidence of bruising/bleeding with or without a history of trauma, further testing of the haemostatic system (Tables 5 & 6) should be undertaken.

References

1. Carpenter RF. The prevalence and distribution of bruising in babies. *Arch Dis Child* 1999; **80**: 363–366.
2. Sugar NF, Taylor JA, Feldman KW. Bruises in infants and toddlers: those who don't cruise don't bruise. Puget Sound Pediatric Research Network. *Arch Pediatr Adolesc Med* 1999; **153**: 399–403.
3. Labee J, Caouette G. Recent skin injuries in normal children. *Pediatrics* 2001; **108**:

271–276.

4. Stephenson T. Ageing of bruising in children. *J R Soc Med* 1997; **90**: 312–314.

5. Manno CS. Difficult pediatric diagnosis. Bruising and bleeding. *Pediatr Clin North Am* 1991; **38**: 637–655.

6. Dunstan FD. A scoring system for bruise patterns: a tool for identifying abuse. *Arch Dis Child* 2002; **86**: 330–333.

7. Vora AJ, Makris M. An approach to investigation of easy bruising. *Arch Dis Child* 2001; **84**: 488–491.

8. Bolton-Maggs PHB, Hill FGH. The rarer inherited coagulation disorders: a review. *Blood Rev* 1995; **9**: 65–76.

9. Harley JR. Disorders of coagulation misdiagnosed as non-accidental bruising. *Paediatr Emerg Care* 1997; **13**: 347–349.

10. Johnson CF, Coury DL. Bruising and hemophilia: accident or child abuse? *Child Abuse Neglect* 1988; **12**: 409–415.

11. O'Hare AE, Eden OB. Bleeding disorders and non-accidental injury. *Arch Dis Child* 1984; **59**: 860–864.

12. Hymel K, Abshire T, Luckey D, Jenny C. Coagulopathy in pediatric abusive head trauma. *Pediatrics* 1997; **3**: 371–375.

13. Taylor D. Child abuse and the eye. *Eye* 1999; **13**: 3–10.

14. Mei-Zahav M, Uziel Y, Raz J, Ginot N, Wolach B, Fainmesser P. Convulsions and retinal haemorrhage: should we look further? *Arch Dis Child* 2002; **86**: 334–335.

15. Gayle M, Hered R, Harwood-Nuss A, Kissoon N. Retinal hemorrhage in the young child: a review of the etiology, predisposed conditions and clinical implications. *J Emerg Med* 1995; **13**: 233–239.

16. Shaw NJ, Eden OB. Juvenile chronic myelogenous leukaemia and neurofibromatosis in infancy presenting as ocular hemorrhage. *Pediatr Hematol Oncol* 1989; **6**: 23–26.

17. Anwar R, Miloszeski KJA. Factor XIII deficiency. *Br J Haematol* 1999; **107**: 468–484.

18. Chiaretti A, Pezzotti P, Mestrovic J *et al*. The influence of hemocoagulative disorders on the outcome of children with head injury. *Pediatr Neurosurg* 2001; **34**: 131–137.

19. Russell-Eggitt I, Thompson D, Khair K, Liesner R, Hann I. Hermansky-Pudlak syndrome presenting with subdural haematoma and retinal haemorrhages in infancy. *J R Soc Med* 2000; **93**: 591–592.

20. Nosek-Cenkowska B, Cheang MS, Pizzi NJ *et al*. Bleeding/bruising symptomatology in children with and without bleeding disorders. *Thromb Haemost* 1991; **65**: 237–241.

21. Wheeler DM, Hobbs CJ. Mistakes in diagnosing non-accidental injury: 10 years' experience. *BMJ* 1988; **296**: 1233–1236.

22. Yeowell HN, Pinnell SR. The Ehlers-Danlos syndromes. *Semin Dermatol* 1993; **12**: 229–240.

23. Kaplinsky C, Kenet G, Seligsohn U, Rechavi G. Association between hyperflexibility of the thumb and an unexplained bleeding tendency: is it a rule of the thumb? *Br J Haematol* 1998; **101**: 260–263.

24. Sham RL, Francis CW. Evaluation of mild bleeding disorders and easy bruising. *Blood Rev* 1994; **8**: 98–104.

25. Chalmers EA, Gibson BES. Acquired disorders of haemostasis during childhood. In: Lilleyman J, Hann I, Blanchette V. (eds) *Pediatric Hematology*. London: Churchill Livingstone, 2000; 629–649.

26. Ritter J, Schrappe M. Clinical features and therapy of lymphoblastic leukaemia. In: Lilleyman J, Hann I, Blanchette V. (eds) *Pediatric Hematology*. London: Churchill Livingstone, 2000; 537–563.

27. Chessells JM. Myelodysplastic syndromes. In: Lilleyman J, Hann I, Blanchette V. (eds) *Pediatric Hematology*. London: Churchill Livingstone, 2000; 83–101.

28. Doyle JJ, Freedman MH. Acquired aplastic anaemia. In: Lilleyman J, Hann I, Blanchette V. (eds) *Pediatric Hematology*. London: Churchill Livingstone, 2000; chapter 2.

29. Al-Jefri A, Bussel J, Freedman M. Thrombocytopenia with absent radii: frequency of marrow megakaryocyte progenitors, proliferative characteristics, and megakaryocyte growth and development factor responsiveness. *Pediatr Hematol Oncol* 2000; **17**: 299–306.

30. Freedman MH, Doyle JJ. Inherited bone marrow failure syndromes. In: Lilleyman J, Hann I, Blanchette V. (eds) *Pediatric Hematology*. London: Churchill Livingstone, 2000; 23–49

31. Mullen C, Anderson K, Blaese R. Splenectomy and/or bone marrow transplantation in the management of the Wiskott-Aldrich syndrome: long term follow-up of 62 cases. *Blood* 1993; **10**: 2961–2966.

32. Hardisty RM. Platelet functional disorders. In: Lilleyman J, Hann I, Blanchette V. (eds) *Pediatric Hematology*. London: Churchill Livingstone, 2000; 465–493.

33. George J, Nurden A. Inherited disorders of the platelet membrane: Glanzmann's thrombasthenia and Bernard-Soulier syndrome. In: Colman R, Hirsch J, Marder V Salzman E. (eds) *Hemostasis and Thrombosis*, 4th edn. Philadelphia, PA: Lippincott, 1994; 921–943.

34. Smith OP. Inherited and congenital thrombocytopenia. In: Lilleyman J, Hann I, Blanchette V. (eds) *Pediatric Hematology*. London: Churchill Livingstone, 2000; 419–435.

35. Harrison CN, Baxter B, Khair K, Russell-Eggitt I, Hann I, Liesner R. Hermansky-Pudlak syndrome: infrequent bleeding and first report of Turkish and Pakistani kindreds. *Arch Dis Child* 2002; **86**: 297–301.

36. Harrison P, Robinson MS, Mackie I *et al.* Performance of the platelet function analyzer PFA-100 in testing abnormal primary haemostasis. *Blood Coagul Fibrinolysis* 1999; **10**: 25–31.

37. Liesner R. The management of coagulation disorders in children. *Curr Paediatr* 2003; In press.

38. Federici AB, Mannucci PM. Advances in the genetics and treatment of von Willebrand disease. *Curr Opin Pediatr* 2002; **14**: 23–33.

39. Mannucci PM. Treatment of von Willebrand disease. *Thromb Haemost* 2001; **86**: 149–153.

40. Peyvandi F, Mannucci PM. Rare coagulation disorders. *Thromb Haemost* 1999; **82**: 1207–1214.

41. Ingerslev J, Kristensen H. Clinical picture and treatment strategies in factor VII deficiency. *Haemophilia* 1998; **4**: 689–696.

42. Girolami A, Simioni P, Scarano L *et al.* Hemorrhagic and thrombotic disorders due to factor V deficiencies and abnormalities: an updated classification. *Blood Rev* 1998; **12**: 45–51.

43. Collins PW, Goldman E, Lilley P *et al.* Clinical experience of factor XI deficiency: the role of fresh frozen plasma and factor XI concentrate. *Haemophilia* 1995; **1**: 227–231.

44. Lak M, Keihani M, Elahi F, Peyvandi F, Mannucci PM. Bleeding and thrombosis in 55 patients with inherited afibrinogenaemia. *Br J Haematol* 1999; **107**: 204–206.

45. Favier R, Aoki N, de Moerloose P. Congenital α_2-plasmin inhibitor deficiencies: a review *Br J Haematol* 2001; **114**: 4–10.

46. Minowa H, Takahashi Y, Tanaka T *et al.* Four cases of bleeding diathesis due to congenital plasminogen activator inhibitor-1 deficiency. *Haemostasis* 1999; **29**: 286–291.

47. Sutor AH, von Kries R, Cornelissen EA, McNinch AW, Andrew M. Vitamin K deficiency bleeding (VKDB) in infancy. *Thromb Haemost* 1999; **81**: 456–461.

48. Roberts HR, Stinchcombe TE, Gabriel DA. The dysfibrinogenaemias. *Br J Haematol* 2001; **114**: 249–257.

49. Scott-Timperley L, Haire W. Autoimmune coagulation disorders. *Rheum Dis Clin North America*; 1997; **2**: 411–423.

Steven M. Schwarz

7

Management of feeding disorders in children with developmental disabilities

Successful completion of the basic activities of daily living may prove difficult if not impossible for the child with significant neurodevelopmental disabilities. Disabled children are at increased risk for developing feeding difficulties and secondary nutritional deficiencies, as consequences of compromised oral motor co-ordination, swallowing function and oesophageal motility.[1–4] These problems comprise significant obstacles to growth, prevent the achievement of developmental potential and threaten clinical stability. Feeding and nutritional problems in disabled patients have been well documented, and clinical evidence of malnutrition has been reported in up to 90% of non-ambulatory children with cerebral palsy.[5] Although many complicating factors certainly contribute to this startling and disturbing observation, functional feeding disorders including gastro-oesophageal reflux (GOR), oral motor disco-ordination, swallowing dysfunction and aversive feeding behaviours have been observed in 30–90% of patients with major motor and cognitive disabilities.[6–9] Failure to assess and treat these feeding problems in a timely fashion not only hastens the onset of significant nutrient deficits, but also heightens the incidence of feeding disorder-related complications, increases hospitalisation rates and costs of care, and results in impaired quality of life.[10,11] This chapter addresses the approach to both evaluating and managing feeding disorders in children with neurodevelopmental disabilities. In addition, it considers the consequences of effective interventions on growth and clinical outcomes.

Prof. Steven M. Schwarz MD FAAP FACN

Professor of Paediatrics, State University of New York Downstate Medical Center and Chairman, Department of Paediatrics, Long Island College Hospital, 339 Hicks Street, Brooklyn, NY 11201, USA
Tel: +1 718 780 1146; Fax: +1 718 780 2569; E-mail: sschwarz@bethisraelny.org

Table 1 Classification of feeding disorders

Oropharyngeal dysphagia
- Poor bolus formation
    - Thin liquids
    - Thickened liquids
    - Solids
- Impaired retrograde propulsion
    - Thin liquids
    - Thickened liquids
    - Solids
- Laryngeal penetration (± aspiration)
    - Thin liquids
    - Thickened liquids
- Pharyngo-oesophageal dyskinesia (± aspiration)

Oesophageal dysmotility*
- Apersistalsis (including achalasia)
- Diffuse oesophageal spasm
- 'Nutcracker' oesophagus
- Non-specific motor abnormalities

Gastro-oesophageal reflux
- With aspiration
- Without aspiration

Aversive feeding behaviours
- Behavioural
- Neurological-behavioural
- Sensory-based

*Not reported with increased frequency in children with neurodevelopmental disabilities.

DEFINITION OF FEEDING DISORDERS

Disorders of oral motor co-ordination, swallowing and oesophageal function have been described using a variety of terminologies (Table 1). For the purposes of this discussion, problems of liquid and/or solid oral bolus formation, propulsion and swallowing are defined by the term oropharyngeal dysphagia.[12] This descriptive entity encompasses oral motor functional disorders (*e.g.* abnormalities in sucking, chewing and lingual movement), swallowing disco-ordination with or without laryngeal penetration, and pharyngo-oesophageal dyskinesia. GOR defines the retrograde (*i.e.* cephalad) propulsion of gastric contents into the oesophagus, often associated with delayed oesophageal acid clearance. Events secondary to GOR include laryngeal penetration, nasopharyngeal and tracheal aspiration of the refluxate. Aversive feeding behaviours, seen commonly in children with primary diagnoses of autism or pervasive developmental delay, include behavioural disorders that are neither structurally nor solely neurologically founded, as well as sensory-based feeding problems. These neurobehavioural disorders involve food refusal unrelated to oropharyngeal dysphagia or GOR.

CLINICAL PRESENTATION

Children with neurodevelopmental disabilities who manifest feeding and nutritional problems may be sub-divided into two broad diagnostic groups.

The first diagnostic category comprises patients who demonstrate significant gross motor dysfunction (often associated with cognitive deficits), with the largest number of children assigned the diagnosis of idiopathic cerebral palsy-mental retardation. Nutritional deficiencies in these patients are commonly associated with poor oral motor co-ordination and swallowing disorders. Accordingly, oropharyngeal dysphagia and GOR represent the most prevalent feeding-related problems.[13] Typical symptoms in affected individuals include excessive drooling leading to ineffective oral feedings with prolonged meal times, coughing or gagging during meals, feeding-associated irritability (secondary to chest pain from oesophagitis) and post-prandial vomiting. Here, complications from feeding disorders include malnutrition as a result of inadequate energy intake, aspiration (secondary to either swallowing dysfunction or to GOR), oesophagitis with or without upper gastrointestinal tract bleeding and oesophageal stricture formation. GOR-related reactive airway disease may develop secondary to micro-aspiration of gastric contents. Experimental data in an animal model also suggest that altered pulmonary function may result from a reflexive increase in airway resistance secondary to GOR without tracheal aspiration of acid.[14] Children in the second major diagnostic group of disabilities usually manifest minor or no gross motor deficits, with autism and pervasive developmental delay representing the most common primary diagnoses. Feeding and nutritional problems in these patients are often the consequences of behavioural food refusal or sensory-based textural aversions. In both patient groups, macro- and micronutrient deficiencies have been reported, although significant clinical evidence of malnutrition is more common in children with severe motor impairments.[1]

EVALUATION AND MANAGEMENT

SCOPE OF THE PROBLEM

As stated previously, feeding and nutritional problems are common complications in developmentally disabled children. Recently, prospective data were collected from 13,971 births enrolled in the Avon (UK) Longitudinal Study of Parents and Children.[15] For 33 infants in this series who subsequently were diagnosed with cerebral palsy, a weak suck was reported at 4 weeks of age in nearly 50%, and significant feeding difficulties were reported at 6 months in 10% of infants. Interestingly, feeding problems at 4 weeks were highly predictive for subsequent swallowing dysfunction and undernutrition by 4–8 years of age. In a review of the Oxford (UK) Register of Early Childhood Impairments, 93% of children with disabilities carried a diagnosis of cerebral palsy and nearly 50% were non-ambulatory.[8] These children with moderate-to-severe neurodevelopmental disabilities commonly manifested feeding problems. Thus, persistent vomiting was described in 22%, choking with feeds occurred in 56% and prolonged feeding times were reported in 28% of affected children. In this review, parents and other caregivers used adjectives such as stressful and unenjoyable to describe mealtimes.

IMPORTANCE OF EARLY INTERVENTION

Follow-up studies clearly demonstrate that early-onset feeding problems in disabled patients represent poor prognostic indicators for the subsequent ability to self-feed effectively. As a consequence, feeding difficulties that commence during infancy are associated with subsequent growth failure and are predictive for adverse developmental outcomes.[15,16] When these problems are recognised early in life, prompt evaluation, diagnosis and nutritional intervention may avoid secondary feeding-associated complications and may maximise growth potential. For example, in one study of 51 children with cerebral palsy, linear growth responses to supplemental tube feedings were greatest when nutritional intervention commenced within 6 months of the primary neurological insult.[17] In children for whom nutritional rehabilitation began after 8 years of age, linear growth remained depressed, although significant weight gain was achieved after instituting a supplemental feeding programme.

DIAGNOSTIC AND THERAPEUTIC APPROACHES

Malnutrition in children with neurodevelopmental disabilities often arises insidiously and is progressive over time. Therefore, assessments of diet and nutritional status for at-risk patients should be should be carried out monthly during the first year of life and at least yearly thereafter (provided, of course, no problems are identified earlier). Feeding and dietary patterns should also be addressed during each routine healthcare visit, and interval histories should include information regarding the duration of mealtimes, presence of feeding-related symptoms and, in toddlers and older children, the development of any specific food preferences or aversions. Once a feeding disorder is suspected, previous studies have shown that an aggressive diagnostic and therapeutic approach to these problems will offer the greatest likelihood to prevent significant malnutrition and to effect successful nutritional rehabilitation.[13,18–20] A multidisciplinary team approach should involve physicians, nurses, behavioural specialists, speech-language pathologists, feeding therapists and parents as care-givers, in order to increase the potential for improved clinical outcomes.

Nutritional assessment

We recently reported our experiences in evaluating and treating a group of 79 children with moderate-to-severe developmental disabilities, who were referred for management of feeding problems.[13] Similar to previously published investigations, the severity of malnutrition in these children correlated with their degree of neurodevelopmental impairment. The most severely compromised patients were non-ambulatory and they manifested varying degrees of spasticity associated with either diplegia or quadriplegia. Clinical assessments of these children suggested a lack of adequate subcutaneous tissue stores, while additional anthropometric measurements demonstrated evidence of chronic malnutrition. Overall nutritional status was evaluated by calculating Z-scores for weight and height. The Z-score is defined by Equation 1:

$$Z = (x - X)/\sigma \qquad \text{Eq. 1}$$

where x equals the patient's weight or height measurement, X equals the age-specific population mean value derived from US National Center for Health Statistics (NCHS) data, and σ represents the standard deviation for the particular measurement and cohort (again, obtained from NCHS figures). While Z-scores indicate relative nutritional status compared to age-matched population norms, triceps and subscapular skin-fold thickness measurements are utilised to determine fat and lean body mass, in order to estimate body composition and gauge the short-term effects of nutritional management. Additional screening studies include determinations of circulating micronutrient levels, especially calcium, phosphorus and vitamin D. Recent evidence indicates that intake of these micronutrients may be inadequate and contributes to osteopenia and pathological fractures in non-ambulatory children.[21] This nutritional assessment information is then used to estimate specific energy requirements (see below) and plan the course of nutritional rehabilitation.

Diagnostic and treatment algorithm

In our published series of disabled children referred for feeding and nutritional assessments,[13] GOR was the most prevalent feeding disorder and affected 56% of subjects. This finding is consistent with previously published data in disabled children and adults, where rates of pathological GOR as high as 70% have been reported.[22,23] Videofluoroscopic swallowing studies demonstrated abnormal swallowing kinetics (*i.e.* oropharyngeal dysphagia) in 26% of our patients. All children in this series who exhibited these functional feeding disorders also manifested significant motor disabilities. Finally, 18% of children in this patient cohort presented for evaluation and management of aversive feeding behaviours. No patient in this diagnostic group (pervasive developmental delay was the most common primary diagnosis) suffered disabling motor abnormalities, and all children demonstrated normal swallowing and gastro-oesophageal function. Based upon these data, an algorithmic model for evaluating and managing feeding disorders in developmentally disabled children has been proposed (Fig. 1). This approach will be discussed in the context of describing specific therapeutic alternatives.

Following completion of the initial history and dietary assessment, children with suspected aversive feeding behaviours and without a clinical suspicion for GOR are evaluated by a trained speech-language pathologist. Observation of feeding patterns and identification of any behavioural and sensory-based solid/liquid or textural preferences will help identify problems with swallowing function that might indicate the need for additional diagnostic studies. If swallowing problems are suspected during the initial speech-language evaluation, a videofluoroscopic swallowing study (VFSS, also referred to as the modified barium swallow) is employed to 'view' swallowing kinetics, assess mechanisms of solid and liquid bolus formation and retrograde bolus propulsion. The VFSS will determine whether the airway is 'protected' against aspiration, identify problems related to swallowing thin versus. thickened liquids and, where indicated, assess difficulties with solid food intake. We perform this study in most children with moderate-to-severe disabilities who are referred for feeding and nutritional evaluations. The VFSS is especially important for patients who are non-ambulatory or who manifest signs of progressive supranuclear palsy, since 'silent' aspiration of thin and/or thickened liquids is a common finding in these patients.[7,24] This study also provides some information regarding oesophageal peristalsis, although dysmotility syndromes (Table 1) and delayed oesophageal clearance (except as a consequence of GOR) have not been reported with great frequency in neurodevelopmentally impaired children. A recently described procedure that employs fibre-optic endoscopy to evaluate swallowing function in paediatric patients may contribute to our diagnostic capabilities without requiring X-ray exposure.[25] Should the swallowing study demonstrate oropharyngeal aspiration, primary endoscopic placement of a gastrostomy tube is generally indicated. Exceptions to this treatment plan include laryngeal aspiration for thin liquids only with normal thickened liquid swallowing kinetics, as well as

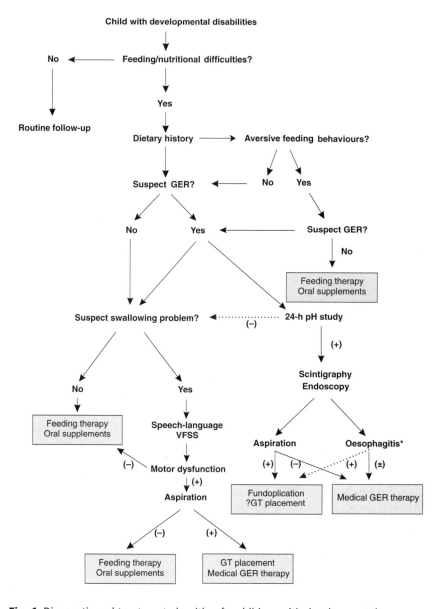

Fig. 1 Diagnostic and treatment algorithm for children with developmental disabilities and feeding problems. *Fundoplication recommended for grade II–IV oesophagitis (see text). Modified from Schwarz *et al.*[13]

evidence of laryngeal penetration that is dependent upon feeding position. Here, appropriate guidance with respect to diet and feeding technique, together with feeding therapy (usually conducted on a weekly or twice per week basis) will significantly reduce the risk for aspiration. In those cases with oropharyngeal dysphagia where oral feedings are maintained, close follow-up is required in order to screen for any subsequent deterioration in oral motor co-ordination, heralding the need for gastrostomy placement. On the other hand, for some malnourished patients whose oral intake is initially limited to thickened formula, improved nutritional status and on-going feeding therapy may result in improved swallowing function for thin liquids (unpublished observation).

Our data and the findings of other groups have confirmed the high incidence of GOR in this patient cohort, and fundoplication is indicated if the milk scinitiscan demonstrates GOR-related aspiration. Anti-reflux surgery is usually recommended when biopsy evidence of moderate to severe oesophagitis (Hill's grade II–IV)[26] is identified during the evaluation for GOR or at the time of endoscopic gastrostomy placement. Even for the patient with oesophagitis, however, intensive nutritional support and a pharmacological trial of acid blockade (either H_2-receptor antagonists or proton pump inhibitors) are warranted prior to referring patients for fundoplication. In fact, one study demonstrated a significant, objective improvement in GOR, evaluated by pH monitoring, following nutritional rehabilitation of disabled children.[27] Other reports have suggested that gastrostomy placement, *per se*, may be associated with development or exacerbation of GOR.[28,29] However, recent studies have refuted this argument,[30,31] and, in our prospective series, no patient who received a gastrostomy alone (without fundoplication) required anti-reflux surgery during a 2-year follow-up period.[13] For children without a clinical history suggesting GOR and without evidence of aspiration during the VFSS, oral nutritional supplements, using defined formula diets, may be sufficient intervention to improve nutritional status. Management of aversive feeding behaviours will also require feeding therapy directed at overcoming food refusal, treating sensory-based eating disorders and assuring adequate nutrient intake. Because of its significance in neurodevelopmentally disabled children, GOR should be considered with a high index of suspicion, including in patients with oral motor problems and without complaints of vomiting, as well as for children with aversive feeding behaviours that may result from subclinical reflux with secondary oesophagitis. Where indicated, evaluations of GOR should comprise 24-h intra-oesophageal pH monitoring, oesophagogastroduodenoscopy, and [99]technetium-sulphur colloid milk scintigraphy to detect aspiration. As stated above, fundoplication will be absolutely required as first-line therapy only for those patients who demonstrate GOR-associated aspiration, and surgery is usually recommended for children manifesting moderate-to-severe oesophagitis.

MEDICAL MANAGEMENT OF GOR

In all published studies, medical management of GOR includes the use of acid-blocking medications. Both H_2-receptor antagonists and proton pump inhibitors may effect some increase in lower oesophageal sphincter tone, mediated via the trophic effects of increased circulating gastrin levels following inhibition of the acid-regulated gastrin negative feedback loop. However, the primary pharmacological effects of these agents involve reduced gastric hydrochloric acid secretion, and their major therapeutic role is clearly to prevent acid-induced oesophageal injury and accelerate healing of oesophagitis. Currently, major controversies surround the indications and use of prokinetic drugs for the treatment of GOR. Prior to the introduction of cisapride, urecholine (Bethanacol) and metoclopramide (Reglan) were the most commonly used prokinetics. Although both drugs appear to reduce the frequency and duration of GOR episodes during pH monitoring, no clear evidence supports their clinical superiority to conservative management and gastric acid reduction. Until its recent withdrawal from the domestic market, cisapride (Propulsid) was the most widely prescribed prokinetic agent used for management of GOR associated disease (GORD) in the US. This prokinetic agent exerts gastrointestinal motility changes that are mediated via $5-HT_4$ receptors and/or enhanced release of acetylcholine. In 1999, a position paper by the European Society of Paediatric Gastroenterology, Hepatology and Nutrition reviewed available safety and efficacy data and concluded that cisapride was the most effective prokinetic agent studied to date, with a wide safety profile across all age groups.[32] Conversely, a recent, systematic review of the drug challenged the validity of these clinical trials.[33] Thus, while cisapride does appear to reduce the reflux index (*i.e.* the percentage time of pH less than 4) during pH monitoring, convincing evidence that supports its clinical effectiveness is lacking. In any case, because of concerns regarding its potential cardiotoxicity (limited, to date, to identifiable at-risk patients), the drug is largely unavailable in the US, except on a compassionate use basis. Future studies will certainly focus on the use of erythromycin for management of GOR, particularly when reflux is associated with prolonged gastric emptying times. Erythromycin is a macrolide antibiotic that exerts influences on the gastrointestinal tract as a motilin receptor agonist, when used in sub-antimicrobial doses, and both animal and human studies have demonstrated its prokinetic effect. Although few paediatric studies have been conducted, evidence has shown beneficial effects of erythromycin in improving tolerance to enteral feedings or enhancing motility. Further studies are eagerly awaited that will identify and evaluate this agent and other, newer approaches for medical management of refractory GOR.

NUTRITIONAL REQUIREMENTS

By following the decision tree suggested in Figure 1, diagnosis-specific interventions will limit the occurrence of feeding-associated complications and offer the greatest opportunity for achieving nutritional rehabilitation. Although feeding disorders represent significant barriers to improving long-term clinical outcomes for disabled children, well-established diagnostic and therapeutic methods are available to evaluate and treat both behavioural and neurological–structural problems. After developing strategies for addressing functional and behavioural feeding disorders, optimal management of children with disabilities depends upon accurately determining nutritional requirements. However, conventional mathematical formulae for estimating steady-state energy expenditure, including the Harris-Benedict and World Health Organization equations, may be inaccurate in this clinical setting. These equations are based upon the age, gender, weight and height of developmentally normal subjects, and they often overestimate energy expenditure in disabled patients, particularly those who are non-ambulatory.[4,34] For example, prior studies have shown that the mean ratio between total energy expenditure and resting energy expenditure (TEE:REE) in children and adolescents with spastic quadriplegia is significantly lower than the mean ratio in normal controls. The TEE:REE ratio is also lower in adequately nourished quadriplegic children than the average value in poorly nourished subjects manifesting similar neurodevelopmental disabilities.[4] Certainly, both dietary and non-dietary influences, including inadequate calorie intake and physical immobility, may contribute to reduced energy expenditure and nutrient deficiencies in the most severely impaired, non-ambulatory patients.[35,36] These problems may be even more complex in nutritionally growth-stunted children, where evidence suggests that endogenous fat oxidation is impaired.[36] Therefore, after instituting effective management strategies to treat feeding disorders, reduced steady-state energy expenditure of growth impaired, non-ambulatory children may actually increase the likelihood of excessive weight gain and subsequent obesity.[36]

To account for the unique problems related to estimating nutritional requirements in non-ambulatory subjects, prior studies have proposed modified calculations of energy requirements. Corrected estimates of basal metabolic rates or the recommended daily allowance (RDA) for energy intake provided by the US National Research Council (for patients without disabling motor impairments) consider factors such as muscle tone, movement and activity to determine requirements for non-ambulatory patients.[37–39] Newer equations for predicting energy expenditure, based upon estimates of fat-free body mass derived from skin-fold thickness measurements, have recently been proposed for non-ambulatory, adult patients.[34] These equations have not yet been evaluated in a disabled paediatric population.

OUTCOMES

Few available studies have examined long-term clinical outcomes of nutritional intervention for children with neurodevelopmental disabilities. Investigations in disabled adult patients have shown that management strategies aimed at reducing complications from swallowing disorders may be life-sustaining. Thus, in one recent report, unadjusted Kaplan-Meier curves indicated that institutionalised patients with feeding tubes were significantly ($P < 0.001$) less likely to die than were subjects without feeding tubes, when followed for 2 years.[40] For children with neurodevelopmental disabilities, goals of nutritional management should include improving nutritional status, reducing feeding-related complications, decreasing costs of care and, where feasible, maximising overall level of functioning. Previous work has demonstrated that motor and cognitively impaired children who receive comprehensive, multidisciplinary nutritional services are adequately nourished and achieve nutritional intakes that meet estimated requirements.[17] In severely disabled children with cerebral palsy and oropharyngeal dysphagia, care-giver interview data suggest that tube feedings improve quality-of-life indicators, both for the child and for the family.[41] Conversely, gastrostomy tube feedings have been associated with late complications, including extruded or 'buried' tubes, gastric metaplasia adjacent to the gastrostomy tube site, and gastric mucosal ulceration.[42] These problems should be considered when contemplating gastrostomy tube insertion; nevertheless, in our experience, the benefits gained from assuring adequate nutriture via gastrostomy tube far outweigh the inherent risks from long-term tube insertion. As stated earlier, gastrostomy tube feedings have been shown to decrease the severity of GOR in neurologically impaired children, and they may significantly reduce the need for anti-reflux surgery. Our recent study confirmed the efficacy of gastrostomy tube placement alone for disabled children with swallowing dysfunction, with or without GOR.[13]

Effects on morbidity from malnutrition and feeding disorder-related illness also serve to measure the benefits of nutritional rehabilitation and feeding therapy in disabled children. Problems such as aspiration pneumonia, feeding-associated hypoxaemia, reactive airway disease and bedsores secondary to immobility and nutritional deficiencies significantly increase acute-care hospitalisations and the costs of care. In our recent follow-up study, the acute-care hospitalisation rate decreased from 0.4 hospital admissions per patient-year in the 2 years prior to nutritional intervention, to 0.15 admissions per patient-year over the 2 years following commencement of diagnosis-specific therapy ($P < 0.01$).[13] Based upon an average length of stay of approximately 5 days for children admitted to our hospital (frequently longer for children with developmental disabilities), at least 180 hospital days were saved over a 2-year period, for this group of 79 children. Finally, at a time when costs of care are a major concern for healthcare administrators, management strategies are judged not only by effects on immediate clinical status and long-term morbidity, but also by the impact of diagnostic and treatment protocols on the utilisation of diminishing resources. Accordingly, prompt and appropriate management of feeding disorders in children with neurodevelopmental disabilities not only enhances clinical outcomes and improves quality-of-life measures, but also reduces the financial burdens associated with repeated and prolonged hospitalisations on families, healthcare providers and institutions.

Key points for clinical practice

- Feeding and nutritional disorders are common problems in children with neurodevelopmental disabilities, affecting as many as 90% of non-ambulatory patients.

- In the routine care of infants and children with (or at-risk for) significant motor and/or cognitive disabilities, nutritional evaluations and clinical assessments of feeding should be conducted monthly for the first year of life, and at least yearly thereafter.

- Developmental disabilities characterised by major motor impairments (± cognitive problems) are frequently associated with oral motor disco-ordination, swallowing dysfunction and gastro-oesophageal reflux (GOR).

Key points for clinical practice (continued)

- Developmental disabilities characterised by cognitive dysfunction and without significant motor problems are most frequently associated with sensory-behavioural food aversions.

- Following a structured algorithm for the diagnosis and treatment of feeding disorders increases the likelihood for successful clinical outcomes, while optimal management of these problems involves a multidisciplinary team approach.

- When considering nutritional management of non-ambulatory patients, remember that their energy requirements will usually be lower than energy needs for ambulatory subjects.

- For disabled children with GOR and poor nutritional status, medical therapy plus nutritional rehabilitation may decrease the severity of GOR, thus obviating the need for anti-reflux surgery in many patients.

- For children with GOR, fundoplication is indicated for patients with aspiration, and surgery is generally recommended for patients with moderate-to-severe oesophagitis (grade II–IV).

- Gastrostomy tube insertion is indicated for children with aspiration of both thin and thickened liquids that occurs as a consequence of oropharyngeal dysphagia.

- Following gastrostomy placement, swallowing studies should be periodically conducted, since nutritional rehabilitation may lead to improved swallowing function and herald the opportunity to re-establish some oral feedings.

- Diagnosis-specific management of feeding disorders in children with developmental disabilities is associated with improved nutritional status, decreased frequency of feeding-associated complications, better quality-of-life for patients and care-givers, and reduced rates of acute care hospitalisation.

References

1. Dahl M, Thommessen M, Rasmussen M, Selberg T. Feeding and nutritional characteristics in children with moderate or severe cerebral palsy. *Acta Paediatr* 1996; **6**: 697–701.
2. Reilly S, Skuse D, Poblete X. Prevalence of feeding problems and oral motor dysfunction in children with cerebral palsy: a community survey, *J Pediatr* 1996; **6**: 877–882.
3. Gisel EG, Birnbaum R, Schwartz S. Feeding impairments in children: diagnosis and effective intervention. *Int J Orofacial Myology* 1998; **24**: 27–33.
4. Stallings VA, Zemel BS, Davies JC, Cronk CE, Charney EB. Energy expenditure of children and adolescents with severe disabilities: a cerebral palsy model. *Am J Clin Nutr* 1996; **4**: 627–634.
5. Rempel GR, Colwell SO, Nelson RP. Growth in children with cerebral palsy fed via gastrostomy. *Pediatrics* 1988; **82**: 857–862.
6. Waterman ET, Koltai PJ, Downey JC, Cacace AT. Swallowing disorders in a population of children with cerebral palsy. *Int J Pediatr Otolaryngol* 1992; **24**: 63–71.

7. Rogors B, Arvedson J, Buck G, Smart P, Msall M. Characteristics of dysphagia in children with cerebral palsy. *Dysphagia* 1994; **9**: 69–73.
8. Sullivan PB, Lambert B, Rose M, Ford-Adams M, Johnson A, Griffiths P. Prevalence and severity of feeding and nutritional problems in children with neurological impairments: Oxford Feeding Study. *Dev Med Child Neurol* 2000; **42**: 674–680.
9. Burklow KA, Phelps AN, Schultz JR, McConnell K, Rudolph C. Classifying complex pediatric feeding disorders. *J Pediatr Gastroenterol Nutr* 1998; **27**: 143–147.
10. Morton RE, Wheatley R, Minford J. Respiratory tract infections due to direct and reflux aspiration in children with severe neurodisability. *Dev Med Child Neurol* 1999; **41**: 329–334.
11. Toder DS. Respiratory problems in the adolescent with developmental delay. *Adolesc Med* 2000; **11**: 617–631.
12. Lefton-Greif MA, Crawford TO, Winkelstein JA *et al*. Oropharyngeal dysphagia and aspiration in patients with ataxia-telangiectasia. *J Pediatr* 2000; **136**: 225–231.
13. Schwarz SM, Corredor J, Fisher-Medina J, Cohen J, Rabinowitz S. Diagnosis and treatment of feeding disorders in children with developmental disabilities. *Pediatrics* 2001; **108**: 671–676.
14. Boyle JT, Tuchman DN, Altschuler SM, Nixon TE, Pack AI, Cohen S. Mechanisms for the association of gastroesophageal reflux and bronchospasm. *Am Rev Respir Dis* 1985; **31**: S16–S20.
15. Motion S, Northstone K, Edmond A, Stucke S, Golding J. Early feeding problems in children with cerebral palsy: weight and neurodevelopmental outcomes. *Dev Med Child Neurol* 2002; **44**: 40–43.
16. Stallings VA, Charney EB, Davies JC, Cronk CE. Nutritional status and growth of children with diplegic or hemiplegic cerebral palsy. *Dev Med Child Neurol* 1993; **35**: 997–1006.
17. Sanders KD, Cox K, Cannon R *et al*. Growth response to enteral feeding by children with cerebral palsy. *J Parenter Enter Nutr* 1990; **14**: 23–26.
18. Pesce KA, Wodarski LA, Wang M. Nutritional status of institutionalized children and adolescents with developmental disabilities. *Res Dev Disabil* 1989; **10**: 33–52.
19. Rogors B, Stratton P, Msall M *et al*. Long-term morbidity and management strategies of tracheal aspiration in adults with severe developmental disabilities. *Am J Ment Retard* 1994; **98**: 490–498.
20. Brant CQ, Stanich P, Ferrari Jr AP. Improvement in children's nutritional status after enteral feeding by PEG: an interim report. *Gastrointest Endosc* 1999; **50**: 183–188.
21. Duncan B, Barton LL, Lloyd J, Marks-Katz M. Dietary considerations in osteopenia in tube-fed nonambulatory children with cerebral palsy. *Clin Pediatr* 1999; **38**: 133–137.
22. Bohmer CJ, Niezen-de Boer MC, Klinkenberg-Knol EC, Deville WL, Nadorp JH, Meuwissen SG. The prevalence of gastroesophageal reflux in institutionalized intellectually disabled individuals. *Am J Gastroenterol* 1999; **94**: 804–810.
23. Puntis JW, Thwaites R, Abel G, Stringer MD. Children with neurological disorders do not always need fundoplication concomitant with percutaneous endoscopic gastrostomy. *Dev Med Child Neurol* 2000; **42**: 97–99.
24. Litvan I, Sastry N, Sonies BC. Characterizing swallowing abnormalities in progressive supranuclear palsy. *Neurology* 1997; **48**: 1654–1662.
25. Hartnick CJ, Hartley BE, Miller C, Willging JP. Pediatric fiberoptic endoscopic evaluation of swallowing. *Ann Otol Rhinol Laryngol* 2000; **109**: 996–999.
26. Hill LD, Kozarek RA, Kraemer SJ *et al*. The gastroesophageal flap valve: *in vitro* and *in vivo* observations. *Gastrointest Endosc* 1996; **44**: 541–547.
27. Lewis D, Khoshoo V, Pencharz PB, Golladay ES. Impact of nutritional rehabilitation on gastroesophageal reflux in neurologically impaired children. *J Pediatr Surg* 1994; **29**: 167–169.
28. Mollitt DL, Golladay ES, Seibert JJ. Symptomatic gastroesophageal reflux following gastrostomy in neurologically impaired patients. *Pediatrics* 1985; **75**: 1124–1126.
29. Berezin S, Schwarz SM, Newman LJ, Halata M. Gastroesophageal reflux secondary to gastrostomy tube placement. *Am J Dis Child* 1986; **140**: 699–701.
30. Borowitz SM, Sutphen JL, Hutcheson RL. Percutaneous endoscopic gastrostomy without an antireflux procedure in neurologically disabled children. *Clin Pediatr* 1997; **36**: 25–29.

31. Puntis JW, Thwaites R, Abel G, Stringer MD. Children with neurological disorders do not always need fundoplication concomitant with percutaneous endoscopic gastrostomy. *Dev Med Child Neurol* 2000; **42**: 97–99.

32. Vandenplas Y, Belli DC, Benatar A *et al.* The role of cisapride in the treatment of pediatric gastroesophageal reflux. *J Pediatr Gastroenterol Nutr* 1999; **28**: 518–528.

33. Bourke B, Drumm B. Cochrane's epitaph for cisapride in childhood gastro-oesophageal reflux. *Arch Dis Child* 2002; **86**: 71–72.

34. Dickerson RN, Brown RO, Gervasio JG, Hak EB, Hak LJ, Williams JE. Measured energy expenditure of tube-fed patients with severe neurodevelopmental disabilities. *J Am Coll Nutr* 1999; **18**: 61–68.

35. Chad KE, McKay HA, Zello GA, Bailey DA, Failkener RA, Snyder RE. Body composition in nutritionally adequate ambulatory and non-ambulatory children with cerebral palsy and a healthy reference group. *Dev Med Child Neurol* 2000; **42**: 334–339.

36. Hoffman DJ, Sawaya AL, Verreschi I, Tucker KL, Roberts SB. Why are nutritionally stunted children at increased risk of obesity? Studies of metabolic rate and fat oxidation in shantytown children from Sao Paulo, Brazil. *Am J Clin Nutr* 2000; **72**: 702–707.

37. National Research Council, Food and Nutrition Board. *Recommended Dietary Allowances*, 10th edn. Washington, DC: National Academy Press, 1989.

38. Cully WJ, Middleton TO. Caloric requirements of mentally retarded children with and without motor dysfunction. *J Pediatr* 1969; **75**: 380–386.

39. Krick J, Murphy PE, Markham JF, Shapiro BK. A proposed formula for calculating energy needs of children with cerebral palsy. *Dev Med Child Neurol* 1992; **34**: 481–487.

40. Rudberg MA, Egleston, BL, Grant MD, Brody JA. Effectiveness of feeding tubes in nursing home residents with swallowing disorders. *J Parenter Enter Nutr* 2000; **24**: 97–102.

41. Smith SW, Camfield C, Camfield P. Living with cerebral palsy and tube feeding: a population-based follow-up study. *J Pediatr* 1999; **135**: 307–310.

42. Mathus-Vliegen, Koning H, Taminiau JAJ, Moorman-Voestermans CGM. Percutaneous endoscopic gastrostomy and gastrojejunostomy in psychomotor retarded subjects: a follow-up covering 106 patient years. *J Pediatr Gastroenterol Nutr* 2001; **33**: 488–494.

Eric I. Felner Perrin C. White

8

Management of diabetic ketoacidosis

Diabetic ketoacidosis (DKA) is a common acute complication of diabetes mellitus. Although potentially life-threatening, it is rarely fatal with proper recognition and treatment. Effective therapy requires knowledge of the pathophysiology of the disorder and the relationships between insulin deficiency, fluid and electrolyte losses, and carbohydrate and fat utilization.

PHYSIOLOGY

Diabetic ketoacidosis is the result of a profound lack of insulin, which produces a severe catabolic state. All of the initial clinical features can be explained by alterations in intermediary metabolism mediated by insulin deficiency combined with counter-regulatory hormone excess. Carbohydrate, protein, and fat metabolism are affected causing hyperglycaemia, dehydration, electrolyte depletion, ketosis, and acidosis.[1-6]

Insulin deficiency has several cellular effects, the most important being decreased activity of the GLUT4 glucose transporter. The ability of glucose to enter most cells is thus decreased, except in the brain, which utilizes a glucose transporter that is not insulin regulated.[7,8] Intracellular glucose levels are low even when hyperglycaemia is present. This leads to secretion of counter-regulatory hormones (epinephrine, cortisol, growth hormone, and glucagon) by the adrenals, pituitary and pancreas in a vain attempt to correct the low

Prof. Eric I. Felner MD (for correspondence)
Assistant Professor of Pediatrics, Section Chief, Pediatric Endocrinology, Department of Pediatrics
SL–37, Tulane University School of Medicine, 1430 Tulane Avenue, New Orleans, LA 70112-2699, USA. Tel: +1 504 588 5375; Fax: +1 504 988–1120; E-mail: efelner@tulane.edu

Prof. Perrin C. White MD
Professor of Pediatrics, Section Chief, Pediatric Endocrinology, Department of Pediatrics, University of Texas Southwestern Medical Center, 5323 Harry Hines Blvd, Dallas, TX 75390-9063, USA
Tel: +1 214 648 3501; Fax: +1 214 648 9772; E-mail: perrin.white@utsouthwestern.edu

intracellular glucose levels. These hormones impair insulin secretion (epinephrine), antagonize insulin's action (epinephrine, cortisol, and growth hormone), and promote glycogenolysis and gluconeogenesis (epinephrine, growth hormone, and cortisol). These effects exacerbate the metabolic decompensation.

Excessive glucose production and impaired glucose utilization combine to cause hyperglycaemia. This leads to glycosuria when the renal threshold of ~10 mmol/l (180 mg/dl) is exceeded. The resultant osmotic diuresis produces polyuria, urinary losses of electrolytes, dehydration, and compensatory polydipsia.

The combination of insulin deficiency and elevated plasma levels of stress hormones also accelerates lipolysis and increases plasma concentrations of total lipids, cholesterol, triglycerides, and free fatty acids. The hormonal interplay of insulin deficiency and glucagon excess shunts free fatty acids into ketone body formation; the rate of formation of these ketone bodies, principally β-hydroxybutyrate and acetoacetate, exceeds the capacity for their peripheral utilization and renal excretion. Acetone, formed by non-enzymatic conversion of acetoacetate, is responsible for a fruity-breath odour. Ketones are excreted in the urine along with cations and this further increases losses of water and electrolytes.

Accumulation of ketoacids results in metabolic acidosis. This stimulates central nervous system (CNS) chemoreceptors, causing hyperventilation that reduces CO_2 and produces a compensatory respiratory alkalosis. Hyperventilation is an effective compensatory mechanism above a pH of ~7.10. More severe acidosis tends to depress the CNS. Decreased intravascular volume and hyperosmolality also contribute to CNS depression.

PRESENTATION

Diabetic ketoacidosis is part of the initial presentation of many (~25%) diabetic children, particularly those under 5 years of age.[9]

The symptoms of DKA include malaise, polyuria, polydipsia, anorexia, nausea, vomiting and/or abdominal pain; these may develop insidiously, especially in patients with new-onset diabetes. Patients invariably have signs of dehydration such as dry mucosa, sunken eyes, prolonged capillary refill, and tachycardia. As dehydration becomes more severe, patients develop orthostatic hypotension or signs of frank shock such as supine hypotension, pallor, mottling, and cool extremities. Ketoacidosis causes hyperventilation, manifested as constant deep breathing (Kussmaul respirations) and a fruity-breath odour. The level of consciousness may vary from awake and alert to drowsiness or coma.

Characteristic laboratory findings of diabetic ketoacidosis include glycosuria, ketonuria, hyperglycaemia (glucose > 16.7 mmol/l [300 mg/dl]), ketonaemia (serum β-hydroxybutyrate > 300 mmol/l or serum ketones strongly positive at greater than 1:2 dilution), and metabolic acidosis (pH < 7.30 and bicarbonate < 18 mmol/l). DKA can be graded as severe (pH < 7.1 and bicarbonate < 5 mmol/l), moderate (pH 7.1–7.2 and bicarbonate 5–10 mmol/l), and mild (pH > 7.2 and bicarbonate 10–15 mmol/l). Serum potassium is often high because intracellular potassium ions are exchanged for extracellular hydrogen ions when the patient is acidotic. These biochemical findings usually allow DKA to be distinguished from dehydration, acidosis and/or coma of other aetiologies, such as hypoglycaemia, uraemia, severe gastroenteritis, acute surgical abdomen, lactic acidosis, ingestion, encephalitis, and intracranial lesions.

Precipitating factors for an episode of DKA should be sought. Infections are frequent precipitants of DKA. Patients with insulin-dependent diabetes are prone to bacterial infections, especially if diabetes is not well controlled.[3] Sites for such infections include the urinary tract, sinuses, skin and subcutaneous tissue, and the lungs. Fever may be absent in an infected patient with DKA if the patient is poorly perfused. It should be kept in mind that physical examinations and chest X-rays are unreliable for diagnosing pneumonias in dehydrated patients. Rales and infiltrates may become apparent with rehydration. Conversely, full blood counts are initially of little diagnostic value because high levels of stress hormones (epinephrine and cortisol) lead to demargination of neutrophils, causing leukocytosis with a 'left shift' to neutrophils and band forms even in the absence of infection.[10]

Psychosocial factors often contribute to risk of DKA. Patients who have recurrent episodes of DKA ('frequent flyers') account for a disproportionate number of admissions; children in this situation are often in poorly supervised environments. A social history should delineate the care arrangements for paediatric patients and the existence of psychosocial stressors that might be exacerbating the situation.[3,11] Compliance with all elements of diabetes management should be determined including insulin dosing, capillary blood glucose testing, and diet. In adolescents or adults, the possibility of ethanol or substance abuse should always be considered.

TREATMENT

DKA should be treated with deliberate speed. A delay of treatment for several hours can be detrimental to the patient. Conversely, the clinician should not attempt to correct dehydration and hyperglycaemia too quickly because this may increase the risk of cerebral oedema (see complications).

Patients in DKA should be initially managed in the emergency room, intensive care unit or equivalent setting until they are haemodynamically stable and their metabolic acidosis is resolving. Mannitol (see complications) should be readily available.

MONITORING

Clinical and laboratory parameters should be frequently monitored with careful attention to trends. An accurate and frequently up-dated progress record (Fig. 1) enables any health professional involved with the patient to become quickly familiar with the treatment given and the response to therapy.

Vital signs and mental status should be assessed at least hourly, and the patient should be on a cardiac monitor. Because treatment of DKA involves many hours of fluid administration and blood sampling, it is preferable to establish separate intravenous access sites for these procedures.

An initial blood sample should be sent for venous blood gas, electrolytes (sodium, potassium, chloride, and bicarbonate), serum glucose, urea, creatinine,

Patient weight _____ kg
Maintenance Fluid _____ cc/hr
2.5 × Maintenance Fluid _____ cc/hr

Date	Signs			Serum				Urine		Fluids				
	Vital Signs	Mental Status	Glucose	VBG	Lytes BUN/Cr	Ca/Mg/ Phos	Ketones	Volume (cc)	Ket/Glu	NS (cc)	Insulin __U/cc (cc/hr)	Fluid #1 Without Dextrose (cc/hr) ___ meq KCl/L ___ meq K₃PO₄/L	Fluid #2 With Dextrose (cc/hr) ___ meq KCl/L ___ meq K₃PO₄/L	Total Fluid (cc/hr)

Fig. 1 Diabetic ketoacidosis progress record

calcium, phosphorus, magnesium, serum ketones (β-hydroxybutyrate), and haemoglobin A1c or glycosylated haemoglobin.

Once the diagnosis of DKA has been established and initial laboratory studies have been collected, frequent laboratory monitoring will help guide DKA therapy (Table 1). Serum glucose levels should be followed hourly with laboratory determinations and with a hand-held meter until the two are correlated within 15%. Depending on the linear range of the meter, this generally occurs when the serum glucose is < 22.2 mmol/l (400 mg/dl). Once they correlate, serum glucose may be measured by the laboratory every 4 h and the capillary glucose measured hourly until the insulin delivery is changed from an intravenous to a subcutaneous route.

In cases of severe DKA, the venous blood gas should be measured every 2 h until the pH is 7.2, every 4 h until the pH is 7.3, and discontinued once the pH is greater than 7.3 and the patient is clinically stable. Electrolytes, calcium, phosphorus, and magnesium should be measured every 4 h. If available, a hand-held chemistry meter (*e.g.* i-STAT Corporation) permits rapid bedside monitoring of glucose, pH, electrolytes and calcium.

Table 1 Laboratory sampling during diabetic ketoacidosis therapy

Laboratory parameter	Frequency
Serum glucose	Every hour until correlates with capillary glucose
Capillary glucose	Every hour until off intravenous insulin
Venous blood gas	Every hour during severe DKA, Every 2 h for pH 7.1–7.19, Every 4 h for pH 7.2–7.29
Electrolytes	Every 2 h during severe DKA or hypo- or hyperkalaemia, Then every 4 h
Calcium, magnesium, & phosphorus	Every 4 h
Serum ketones	Every 4 h
Urine ketones/glucose	Every void

In following the electrolytes, the measured sodium concentration should be corrected for the degree of hyperglycaemia because the osmotic fluid shifts due to hyperglycaemia decrease the measured serum sodium. Thus, serum sodium should increase with correction of hyperglycaemia (glucose concentration in mg/dl) according to Equation 1:

$$\text{Corrected } [Na^+] = \text{Measured } [Na^+] + 1.6([glucose]-100)/100 \qquad \text{Eq. 1}$$

Serum β-hydroxybutyrate may be measured every 4 h although it usually adds little to pH or CO_2 levels in monitoring resolution of DKA. Urinary ketones should be measured with each void. Because urinary ketones are measured using a nitroprusside test, significant levels of acetoacetate and acetone are measured in addition to β-hydroxybutyrate. For this reason, and also because urine may be held in the bladder for some time, patients may have resolution of ketonaemia but still have detectable urinary ketones.[12,13] Measurement of urinary ketones should continue until the test is negative to determine when fluid therapy can be discontinued.

FLUID REPLACEMENT

All patients in DKA are dehydrated. Hydration status should be evaluated by such criteria as moisture of mucous membranes and capillary refill time. Patients in DKA are invariably tachycardic, both because of dehydration and because epinephrine levels are increased. Because epinephrine levels may not return to normal until acidosis is resolved, the patient's heart rate may remain elevated despite re-establishment of adequate intravascular volume. Unless dehydration is severe, urine output may remain brisk due to osmotic diuresis. Although the degree of dehydration can sometimes be estimated by comparing the patient's current weight to a recent healthy weight, this is often not readily available and may not be accurate.

For these reasons, it is best to avoid calculating fluid replacement volumes based on the estimated degree of dehydration. Instead, fluids should be delivered at a total rate of ~2.5 times the patient's maintenance fluid requirement. This rate is recommended because retrospective studies suggest that administration of fluids in excess of 4 $l/m^2/24$ h is associated with an increased risk of cerebral oedema.[14,15] Maintenance fluid requirements are 1.5 $l/m^2/24$ h, and thus 2.5 times the maintenance requirement (3.75 $l/m^2/24$ h) ensures provision of adequate but not excessive fluids.[16] In cases of larger children (weight > 75 kg), the maximum maintenance delivery should be for that of a 75 kg patient.

We discuss the fluid regimen under three categories in the chronological order in which they are administered: initial hydration, insulin therapy, and subsequent fluid replacement. Once all fluid components have been initiated, the patient in DKA should be receiving 3 distinct solutions that are combined (piggyback) into one intravenous site that is separate from the blood-sampling site (Fig. 2).

Initial hydration
The initial hydrating fluid should be isotonic saline (0.9% NaCl), which helps to restore intravascular volume and thus maintains blood pressure and kidney

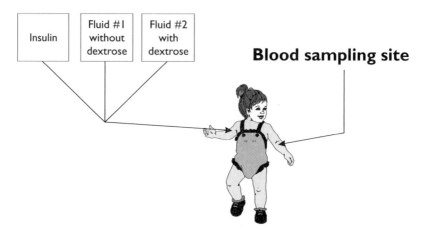

Fig. 2 Fluid delivery and blood sampling during diabetic ketoacidosis therapy.

perfusion. Lactated Ringer's solution is an alternative. Initial hydration increases renal glomerular filtration and thus enhances glucose excretion, decreasing blood glucose levels even before insulin is administered. Due to hyperglycaemia, hyperosmolarity almost invariably occurs in DKA; thus, even 0.9% saline is usually hypotonic relative to the patient's serum osmolarity.

Children should receive an initial bolus (20 ml/kg) of 0.9% sodium chloride over 30 min. For children with pre-existing cardiac or renal insufficiency, an infusion of 10 ml/kg over 30 min is appropriate. Most children in DKA will require only a single bolus to restore intravascular volume, but a second bolus may be provided if peripheral perfusion remains poor (*e.g.* capillary refill time > 3 s). Rarely, colloid (*e.g.* albumin) is needed for patients in shock. Because tachycardia may persist for hours due to elevated epinephrine levels, persistent tachycardia is not by itself a reason to administer another fluid bolus. Although a patient in moderate-to-severe DKA can appear quite ill, the clinician should resist the temptation to correct dehydration completely with initial fluid boluses. Once peripheral perfusion has been restored and the patient is haemodynamically stable, 0.9% sodium chloride should be delivered at a constant rate that ensures a total fluid delivery rate (0.9% sodium chloride and insulin infusions) of 2.5 times the maintenance requirement. The 0.9% sodium chloride infusion should be continued until the appropriate replacement fluids (see later) arrive (1–2 h).

Insulin therapy

A continuous intravenous insulin infusion eliminates the problem of unreliable absorption from subcutaneous sites in a dehydrated patient.[17] Because intravenous insulin is rapidly cleared from the circulation, doses may be adjusted easily and rapidly.

A typical infusion rate for insulin is 0.1 units (U)/kg/h. A loading dose is not necessary. Regular insulin (50 U) is mixed in 250 ml of saline (0.2 U/ml) so that small adjustments in insulin delivery can be made easily. Insulin should be delivered via a separate infusion pump so that the rate can be adjusted independently of other intravenous fluids. When fluids containing glucose are being administered (see below), it is prudent to deliver the insulin and glucose solutions through a Y-connector into the same intravenous catheter, as otherwise loss of the line through which glucose was being infused might result in hypoglycaemia.

Because insulin is required to resolve acidosis, the insulin infusion rate should remain at or above 0.1 U/kg/h until resolution of acidosis. If no improvement in acidosis has occurred within a few hours of insulin therapy, the insulin rate should be increased by 0.05 U/kg/h every 2 h, until acidosis begins to improve; it is very unusual that this requires a rate exceeding 0.2 U/kg/h. In general, rather than decreasing the rate of insulin infusion, an excessively rapid fall in blood glucose should be treated by increasing the rate of dextrose delivery. Interruptions in the insulin infusion, if they occur, should be limited to a few minutes because acidosis can quickly worsen in the absence of insulin.

Subsequent fluid replacement

In response to fluids and insulin, patients will often normalize their glucose levels in less than half the time it takes to resolve the acidosis.[18] Since the end-point of DKA treatment is resolution of acidosis, glucose must be infused to control the rate of decrease of blood glucose and prevent hypoglycaemia. The rate at which blood glucose falls is a function of the rates at which both insulin and glucose are infused. It is useful to conceptualize this as a ratio of grams of glucose to units of insulin infused. If the blood glucose level drops by more than 5.6 mmol/l/h (100 mg/dl/h), more than 19.4 mmol/l (350 mg/dl) in 6 h, or when the glucose level falls below 16.7 mmol/l (300 mg/dl), a glucose infusion should be started. A typical initial rate is 3–4 g of glucose/unit of insulin being infused. This can be subsequently modified to produce a rate of decrease of blood glucose of ~2.8 mmol/l/h (50 mg/dl/h) to a level of ~8.3 mmol/l (150 mg/dl), which should be maintained for the duration of DKA treatment.

In principle, the glucose:insulin ratio could be modified by varying the rate of the insulin infusion or the rate of a single glucose-containing intravenous solution. However, it is preferable to maintain constant rates of insulin and total fluid infusions to ensure steady improvement in acidosis. Although fluids with different concentrations of glucose could be ordered, this is expensive and cumbersome; it may engender treatment delays if new fluids are not provided in a timely manner by the pharmacy.

Therefore, it is preferable to order two separate solutions that are identical in electrolyte composition; one contains glucose (10 g/dl of dextrose) and the other does not.[16,19] The total rate of infusion of the two fluids is held constant at ~2 times the maintenance fluid rate, and the rate of each solution varied to yield the desired glucose infusion rate.

For example, a 30 kg child (~1 m² body surface area) would have a main-tenance fluid rate of 1500 ml/24 h, so that the two solutions should be infused at a total rate of 3000 ml/24 h or 125 ml/h. Insulin would be infused at 3 units/h. If a 3:1 glucose:insulin ratio were desired, this would require 9 g/h of

Table 2 Potassium and phosphate replacement during diabetic ketoacidosis therapy

Serum potassium (meq/l)	Amount of KCl to add (meq/l)	Amount of K_2HPO_4 to add (meq/l)
< 4.0	30	30
4.0–5.5	20	20
> 5.5	0*	0*

*Order dextrose and non-dextrose solutions with 20 meq KCl/l and 20 meq K_2HPO_4/l. Do not infuse until potassium level is < 5.6 meq/l.

glucose, or 90 ml/h of a 10 g/dl solution. Therefore, the solution without glucose would be infused at 35 ml/h.

Sodium

Due to osmotic diuresis, patients in DKA are depleted of sodium upon presentation. They usually require ~20 mmol/kg of NaCl over the first 24 h of treatment. Although many protocols recommend intravenous fluids containing 0.45% NaCl (75 mmol/l), this may not provide adequate sodium replacement at recommended fluid rates. Therefore, intravenous fluids should contain 0.675% NaCl (115 mmol/l). This will usually limit the decrease in serum sodium to ~5 mmol/l over the first 24 h of treatment. If hypernatraemia or hyperchloraemic acidosis supervenes, the NaCl concentration can be decreased to 0.45%. Conversely, the sodium concentration can be increased if the corrected serum sodium decreases by > 10 mmol/l within the first 12 h of treatment.

Potassium

Patients with DKA invariably have significant total-body potassium depletion, but serum potassium is usually high or normal upon presentation. Treatment with insulin causes potassium to move intracellularly, rapidly decreasing serum potassium. Potassium should be infused when the serum potassium level is < 5.6 mmol/l and the patient is voiding. Usually a total of 40 mmol/l of potassium is added to intravenous fluids, half as potassium chloride and half as potassium phosphate (see Table 2). Because of the rapid decrease in potassium levels with insulin therapy and the time lag associated with receiving fluids from many hospital pharmacies, it is prudent to order fluids containing potassium at the time the diagnosis is established. These may be held in reserve until the serum potassium falls to safe levels.

Sodium bicarbonate

Although sodium bicarbonate is administered to treat other forms of acidosis, it is rarely necessary in patients with DKA. Patients will gradually correct their acidosis as insulin and fluid treatment proceed and ketone bodies are metabolized or excreted. The rate in recovery is equal in patients treated with and without bicarbonate. The potential risks of bicarbonate include rebounding metabolic alkalosis, paradoxical cerebrospinal fluid acidosis, impaired tissue oxygenation, and worsening of hypokalaemia. The use of bicarbonate is associated with an increased risk for developing cerebral oedema.[20]

In patients who are severely acidotic (pH < 7.0) and in poor clinical condition (*i.e.* shock, acute renal failure, or symptomatic hyperkalaemia) a single small dose of bicarbonate (1 mmol/kg/dose over 30 min, maximum dose 50 mmol) may improve myocardial contractility and prevent further CNS depression.

DKA TREATMENT IN A MEDICALLY UNDERSERVED AREA

The preceding discussion assumes availability of infusion pumps that can deliver precise volumes, a laboratory that can measure blood gases and serum electrolytes quickly, and a pharmacy that can provide appropriate intravenous fluids. Compromises obviously must be made if one or more of these are not available.

If there are no satisfactory infusion pumps, fluids can be administered at the recommended rates by drip infusion. Regular or, preferably, Lispro insulin may be administered by intramuscular injection every 1–2 h at the recommended rate of 0.1 U/kg/h. Subcutaneous injections should be avoided in a dehydrated patient because absorbtion is unpredictable and there is a risk of late hypoglycaemia as insulin is flushed into the circulation with improved hydration.

If there is no pharmacy on site, combinations of standard intravenous fluids (*e.g.* 10% dextrose with 0.45% NaCl) may be used as long as potassium is added to yield the recommended concentrations. The frequency of laboratory monitoring should be maintained to the extent possible, particularly as regards blood or serum glucose and electrolyte determinations.

CONVERTING TO SUBCUTANEOUS INSULIN

Patients should be continued on intravenous insulin until they are haemodynamically stable, have resolved their acidosis, are alert, and can take fluids and food orally without vomiting. This usually takes 12–14 h. It is most convenient to switch from intravenous insulin to subcutaneous insulin at the next regular meal (*i.e.* breakfast, lunch, or supper). If the patient has established diabetes, the previous home regimen should be followed. If the patient is newly diagnosed, a subcutaneous insulin regimen should be established that the patient could be taught to use at home. A detailed discussion of home insulin regimens is beyond the scope of this chapter. In general, the recommendations of the Diabetes Control and Complications Trial should be followed, so that patients receive three or four injections over the day.[21] A typical initial insulin regimen for a prepubertal child would include 0.4 U/kg (divided two-thirds NPH and one-third regular or Lispro) before breakfast, 0.1 U/kg of regular or Lispro before supper, and 0.1 U/kg of NPH at bedtime. If the patient is being switched from intravenous to subcutaneous insulin at lunch (a time when the child would not otherwise get an insulin injection), 0.1 U/kg of regular or Lispro insulin may be administered. Once the food arrives, the insulin is injected subcutaneously. If regular insulin is used, the patient may be allowed to eat 20–30 min after the injection; if Lispro is used, the patient may begin eating immediately after the injection. The intravenous glucose and insulin solutions are discontinued at the time the patient is allowed to eat. The intravenous solution without glucose may be continued at the maintenance rate if the patient still has significant ketosis. Once subcutaneous insulin has been injected, the capillary blood glucose should be measured before meals, at bedtime, midnight and 4 a.m. to assist in insulin dose adjustments.

DIAGNOSIS AND TREATMENT OF CEREBRAL OEDEMA

Cerebral oedema is a serious complication of DKA treatment that accounts for half or more of DKA-associated deaths. It usually occurs after 4–12 h of treatment while biochemical abnormalities are improving. Although subclinical brain swelling may be detected by computed tomography or magnetic resonance imaging in many patients with DKA,[22,23] overt cerebral oedema occurs in less than 1% of properly treated patients.[16,20,24] Children younger than 5 years of age and those with new-onset diabetes mellitus make up an excessive proportion of cases. More severe acidosis (or decreased arterial partial pressure of carbon dioxide) and more severe dehydration (or increased serum urea nitrogen) at presentation are also risk factors. Among therapeutic interventions, administration of bicarbonate is associated with increased risk.[20] Whereas a high rate of fluid administration ($> 4 l/m^2/24 h$) has been previously associated with increased risk in retrospective studies,[14,15] neither rate of infusion of fluids nor amount of sodium administered is a risk factor in case-controlled studies in which patients are treated using modern protocols. Among therapeutic responses, rate of decrease in blood glucose is not a risk factor, but falling serum sodium, or failure of serum sodium to increase with treatment, is associated with increased risk.[16,20,24] It is not clear whether this represents a cause or an effect of the pathological processes causing cerebral oedema.

The clinician should be alert for prodromal symptoms and signs of impending cerebral oedema; these occur in approximately half of patients. They include headache, a dilated or unreactive pupil, and deteriorating mental status (irritability, decreased co-operation, disorientation, decreased level of consciousness). Many patients in DKA are initially lethargic, but this usually improves quickly on therapy. Vital signs should be monitored for bradycardia, hypertension and decreased respirations (Cushing's triad). It is important to be aware of the normal heart rate for the patient's age. The heart rate in a patient with DKA should decrease with intravenous fluid therapy and resolution of acidosis, but not to below the normal range. Recrudescence of vomiting is worrisome; most patients in DKA are vomiting on presentation, but this should improve on therapy.

Time is of the essence in treating cerebral oedema; the outcome is often poor if treatment is delayed until respiratory arrest has ensued. If the patient is obtunded, secure the airway and ensure that the patient is breathing. Raise the head of bed 30 degrees and keep the head in the midline. Decrease the intravenous fluid rate to maintenance or less. Administration of mannitol (0.5 g/kg i.v. over 5 min), an osmotic diuretic, is a mainstay of treatment. It is prudent to have mannitol available at the bedside in any patient with severe DKA. One or two additional doses (0.25 g/kg) may be given every 5–10 min until a response (improved level of consciousness, stable vital signs, regaining pupillary response) is obtained. The patient should be hyperventilated. If the patient is obtunded, this may be started immediately with bag and mask, but intubation with paralysis and sedation are more effective. If the patient is sufficiently stable, computed tomography or magnetic resonance imaging of the head should be performed. A neurosurgical consultation should be obtained and intracranial pressure monitoring begun. Patients may occasionally require 24–48 h of hyperventilation, deep sedation and repeated doses of mannitol before intracranial pressure stabilizes.

With current therapy, ~70% of patients will survive cerebral oedema, and approximately two-thirds of survivors will be free of neurological sequelae.

Key points for clinical practice

- Diabetic ketoacidosis (DKA) is a common acute complication of diabetes mellitus, characterized by hyperglycaemia and acidaemia (pH < 7.30).
- Diabetic ketoacidosis is rarely fatal if it is properly recognized and appropriate therapy is initiated.
- The pathophysiology of diabetic ketoacidosis involves both insulin deficiency and elevated levels of counter-regulatory hormones including glucagon, epinephrine and cortisol.
- Precipitating factors should be sought, particularly infections and lack of compliance with diabetes management.
- Signs of infection may be obscured in severely dehydrated patients, and leukocyte counts are usually elevated even in the absence of infection.
- Diabetic ketoacidosis is treated with intravenous fluids and insulin.
- Clinical status (vital signs, mental status, cardiac monitor) must be closely monitored.
- Biochemical parameters that must be closely monitored during treatment include blood glucose, electrolytes and pH.
- The aim of initial fluid resuscitation is restoration of intravascular volume and not complete resolution of dehydration.
- Total fluid delivery should be ~2.5 times the maintenance fluid rate, or < 4 l/m^2/24 h, to treat dehydration while minimizing risk of cerebral oedema.
- Concentrations of sodium and potassium in intravenous fluids must be adequate to prevent hyponatraemia and hypokalaemia.
- Hyperglycaemia usually resolves before acidosis. To resolve acidosis while avoiding hypoglycaemia, intravenous insulin must be continued, and blood glucose maintained with intravenous fluids containing glucose.
- A 3-bag protocol provides an efficient means for independently adjusting glucose delivery while maintaining adequate rates of insulin and fluid delivery.
- Cerebral oedema is a rare but serious complication of diabetic ketoacidosis, the development of which is often heralded by changes in vital signs or mental status.
- To minimize death or permanent sequelae, cerebral oedema must be treated promptly by maintaining an airway, hyper-ventilation, fluid restriction, and intravenous mannitol.

References

1. Menon RK, Sperling MA. Childhood diabetes. *Med Clin North Am* 1988; **72**: 1565–1576.
2. Schade DS, Eaton RR. The temporal relationship between endogenously secreted stress hormones and metabolic decompensation in diabetic man. *J Clin Endocrinol Metab* 1980; **50**: 131–136.
3. Sperling MA. Diabetic ketoacidosis. *Pediatr Clin North Am* 1984; **31**: 591–610.
4. Foster DW, McGarry JD. The metabolic derangements and treatment of diabetic ketoacidosis. *N Engl J Med* 1983; **309**: 159–169.
5. Fleckman AM. Diabetic ketoacidosis. *Endocrinol Metab Clin North Am* 1993; **22**: 181–207.
6. White NH. Diabetic ketoacidosis in children. *Endocrinol Metab Clin North Am* 2000; **29**: 657–682.
7. Devaskar SU, Mueckler NM. The mammalian glucose transporters. *Pediatr Res* 1992; **31**: 1–13.
8. Kahn BB. Facilitative glucose transporters: regulating mechanisms and dysregulation in diabetes. *J Clin Invest* 1992; **89**: 1367–1374.
9. Jefferson IG, Smith MA, Baum JD. Insulin dependent diabetes in under 5 year olds. *Arch Dis Child* 1985; **60**: 1144–1148.
10. Flood RG, Chiang VW. Rate and prediction of infection in children with diabetic ketoacidosis. *Am J Emerg Med* 2001; **19**: 270–273.
11. Keenan HT, Foster CM, Oratton SL. Social factors associated with prolonged hospitalization among diabetic children. *Pediatrics* 2002; **109**: 40–44.
12. Stephens JM, Sulway MJ, Watkins PJ. Relationship of blood acetoacetate and 3-hydroxybutyrate in diabetes. *Diabetes* 1971; **20**: 485–489.
13. Reichard GA, Skutches CL, Hoeldtke RD *et al*. Acetone metabolism in humans during diabetic ketoacidosis. *Diabetes* 1986; **35**: 668–674.
14. Duck SC, Wyatt DT. Factors associated with brain herniation in the treatment of diabetic ketoacidosis. *J Pediatr* 1988; **113**: 10–14.
15. Mahoney CP, Vlcek BW, DelAguila M. Risk factors for developing brain herniation during diabetic ketoacidosis. *Pediatr Neurol* 1999; **21**: 721–727.
16. Felner EI, White PC. Improving management of diabetic ketoacidosis in children. *Pediatrics* 2001; **108**: 735–740.
17. Kaufman IA, Keller MA, Nyhan WL. Diabetic ketosis and acidosis: the continuous infusion of low doses of insulin. *J Pediatr* 1975; **87**: 846–848.
18. Schade DS, Eaton RR. Dose response to insulin in man: differential effects on glucose and ketone body regulation. *J Clin Endocrinol Metab* 1977; **44**: 1038–1053.
19. Grimberg A, Cerri RW, Satin-Smith M, Cohen P. The 'two-bag system' for variable intravenous dextrose and fluid administration: benefits in diabetic ketoacidosis management. *J Pediatr* 1999; **134**: 376–378.
20. Glaser N, Barnett P, McCaslin I *et al*. Risk factors for cerebral edema in children with diabetic ketoacidosis. *N Engl J Med* 2001; **344**: 264–269.
21. The Diabetes Control and Complications Trial Research Group. The effect of intensive treatment of diabetes on the development and progression of long-term complications in insulin-dependent diabetes mellitus. *N Engl J Med* 1993; **329**: 977–986.
22. Krane EJ, Rockoff MA, Wallman JK *et al*. Subclinical brain swelling in children during treatment of diabetic ketoacidosis. *N Engl J Med* 1985; **312**: 1147–1151.
23. Hoffman WH, Casanova MF, Bouza JA, Passmore CG, Sekul EA. Computer analysis of magnetic resonance imaging of the brain in children and adolescents after treatment of diabetic ketoacidosis. *J Diabetes Complications* 1999; **13**: 176–181.
24. Mel JM, Werther GA. Incidence and outcome of diabetic cerebral oedema in childhood: are there predictors? *J Pediatr Child Health* 1995; **31**: 17–20.

Carole Jenny

9

The assessment and management of genital and anal warts

Genital and anal warts in children challenge clinicians with difficult diagnostic and management problems. The epidemiology of these lesions in prepubertal children is not clearly defined, and their possible relationship to sexual contact leaves clinicians with uncomfortable diagnostic dilemmas. None of the topical therapies approved for treatment of external genital and anal warts in adults have been formally tested in children. The long-term significance of early infection with a potentially oncogenic wart virus is unknown. Much of what we presume to know about genital and anal warts in children is information extrapolated from research on similar lesions in adults. This article addresses external warts primarily, and will not address current practice or controversies in the diagnosis and management of cervical dysplasia in adolescent girls.

HUMAN PAPILLOMAVIRUS

AETIOLOGY OF ANAL AND GENITAL WARTS

Human papillomavirus (HPV) is a small, non-enveloped virus consisting of 72 capsomeres with icosahydral symmetry. The virus has an 18 kb circular, double-stranded genome of DNA.[1] At least 28 different types of HPV have been shown to infect the human genital tract. The virus is typed based on its homology with known virus types. In warts, the virus replicates as extrachromosomal episomes within the cell nuclei. Certain types of virus are characterized as 'high-risk' types. These viruses can integrate into the host genome, leading to 'deregulation' of the host DNA. Two HPV genes have been identified that produce oncoproteins that can lead to the development of neoplasia.[2]

Prof. Carole Jenny MD MBA
Professor of Pediatrics, Hasbro Children's Hospital, POB-130, 593 Eddy Street, Providence, RI 02906, USA. Tel: +1 401 444 3996; Fax: +1 401 444 7397; E-mail: cjenny@lifespan.org

The most common 'low-risk' HPVs are types 6 and 11. They are seldom associated with cancerous lesions, and usually cause warts on the vulva, vagina and anus rather than on the cervix. Types 16 and 18 are the most common 'high risk' types of HPV, and are frequently found in invasive cancers.[3]

HPVs cannot infect mature epithelial cells, and must gain access to the basilar cell layers of the epithelium (cells adherent to the basement membrane) to establish infections. This presumably occurs through abrasions or 'microtrauma' on the epithelial surface. Each wart is thought to represent clones of epithelial cells infected with a single virus. As the infected cells push up through the epithelium, viral DNA replication occurs near the surface, leading to the differentiation of cells and production of viral capsids.[4]

CLINICAL MANIFESTATIONS OF EXTERNAL HPV INFECTION

Four morphologies of external anal and genital warts are described. The morphologies appear on different types of anal and genital skin (Table 1).[5] Most flat, macular warts are caused by HPV types 16, 33, or 42 ('high-risk' types), while typical 'cauliflower warts' (condylomata acuminata) are usually caused by types 6 and 11.[4] HPV is found in other types of anal and genital skin lesions as well. Buschke-Löwenstein tumours (giant condylomata) are large, slow-growing, locally invasive lesions that rarely metastasize. Another HPV-related condition, Bowenoid papulosis, has been described in children as well as in adults.[6] These HPV-related lesions are flat-topped, hyperpigmented lesions that resemble melanocytic nevi. Although the lesions are mildly dysplastic, they are unlikely to be invasive and are generally self-limiting.

HPV infections of the skin can be clinically obvious, subclinical or latent. Obvious genital and anal warts are usually diagnosable by visual inspection, although a variety of normal and pathological clinical conditions can be confused with warts (Table 2). If the diagnosis is in question, it can be confirmed by biopsy of the suspect lesion.

Some infections are subclinical, and are not noted on visual inspection. They can be seen by applying 3–5% acetic acid to the epithelium. On external skin, acetic acid should be applied for 3–5 min for whitening to occur.[7] This

Table 1 Skin surface types and associated wart morphology of the external anus and genitals[5]

Skin surface type	Wart morphology
Fully keratinized hair-bearing or non-hair-bearing skin	Keratotic warts with a thick, horny layer resembling common warts
	Smooth, dome-shaped, papular warts 1–4 mm in diameter, usually skin-coloured
	Flat-topped papules that are macular and slightly raised
Partially keratinized, moist, non-hair-bearing skin	Cauliflower-shaped warts (condylomata acuminata)
	Flat-topped papules that are macular and slightly raised

Table 2 Skin lesions that can be misidentified as genital and anal warts[5,15,57–60]

Normal skin variants

        Skin tags
        Epidermal verrucous nevi
        Sebaceous glands
        Pearly penile papules
        Vestibular papillae

Pathological skin conditions

        Congenital lymphangioma circumscriptum
        Acquired lymphangiectasia
        Bowenoid papulosis
        Erythroplasia of Queyrat
        Bowen's disease
        Condylomata lata
        Benign tumours
        Seborrheic keratosis
        Molluscum contagiosum
        Lichen planus
        Lichen niditus
        Psoriasis
        Squamous cell carcinoma
        Fibroma molle
        Pseudoverrucous pappules and nodules
        Vulvar hamartoma
        Eosinophilic granuloma
        Vulvar pemphigus
        Focal epithelial hyperplasia (Heck's disease)
        Histiocytosis X
        Granular cell tumour
        Crohn's disease

coagulates the epithelial cytokeratins causing lesions to appear white ('acetowhitening'). Acetowhitening of lesions of the genitals and anus is not specific for HPV-related lesions, and biopsy of suspicious lesions is required to confirm the diagnosis.[4] Subclinical lesions have been found to be quite common in adults. In one study, 42.5% of partners of women with cervical HPV infections had subclinical penile HPV-related lesions identified with acetowhitening that were not visible before acetic acid was applied.[8]

Latent infection can be found in histologically normal epithelial tissue by identifying the presence of HPV DNA. The latent virus is thought to serve as a reservoir of infection that can lead to recurrence of warts after treatment.[9] Obvious genital and anal warts most likely represent the 'tip of the iceberg' of HPV infection. Of sexually active adults, 1% have clinical genital or anal warts, while 10–20% harbour HPV DNA in the anogenital tissues.[10]

INTRAVAGINAL AND INTRA-ANAL HPV INFECTION

HPV is a potentially oncogenic virus associated with the development of cervical carcinomas and other squamous cell carcinomas. In adolescents, abnormal Papanicolaou (Pap) smears with squamous intra-epithelial lesions are common. In one study, 3.7% of 10–19-year-olds had squamous intra-epithelial lesions, the highest rate in any age group by decade.[11] Squamous intra-epithelial lesions are known to be a risk factor for developing cervical cancer. In addition, the rate of abnormal Pap smears in adolescents has increased dramatically in the past few decades.[12]

Intravaginal and intra-anal HPV infections have been identified in prepubertal girls as well. In a study of 15 Tanner stage I and II sexually abused girls, all under age 12 years, 5 (33%) had HPV isolated from vaginal specimens.[13] Four were typed as HPV type 6 or 11, and one was HPV type 16. Three of the 5 girls had no external genital warts. Four of the 5 HPV positive girls had koilocytosis, atypia, or inflammatory reaction noted on Pap smears obtained from the immature cervixes.

In another study of 18 girls with external genital warts, 8 (44%) had genomic and/or cytological evidence of cervical-vaginal, peri-urethral, or intra-anal HPV infection.[14] These studies suggest that children who experience sexual abuse may be at risk for early acquisition of oncogenic HPV viruses. Sexual abuse in childhood has not been studied in regard to the risk of acquisition of HPV-related cancers in adulthood.

MICROSCOPIC DIAGNOSIS OF HPV INFECTION

On biopsy and cytology,[15] lesions caused by HPV have a characteristic appearance, including:

1. Acanthosis –hypertrophy of the prickle cell layer, the epithelial cell layer found above the basilar cells.

2. Parakeritosis – active HPV infection causes cells in stratum corneum, the most external cell layer of the epithelium, to retain their nuclei. This is referred to as 'parakeritosis'.

3. Hyperkeratosis – hypertrophy of the horny, outside layer of the epidermis.

4. Papillomatosis – elongated dermal papillae, reaching up toward the surface of the epithelium.

5. Dyskeratosis – defective keratin formation where the cells of the epidermis form keratin prematurely, in lower cell layers of the epithelium than normal.

6. Multinuclear cells – cells with more than one nuclei.

7. Koilocytes – cells with a dark, pyknotic nuclei surrounded by a clear cytoplasmic ring caused by cytoplasmic degeneration. The nuclei are enlarged and have an irregular border.

Not all HPV-positive tissue will have these typical histological changes. Some will manifest no changes, and others will have some or all of the above characteristics present. Koilocytosis is considered the most specific diagnostic cytological finding indicating HPV infection, but it is not a sensitive or specific predictor of the presence of HPV.[16]

TESTING FOR HPV DNA

HPV cannot be grown in clinical laboratories for identification purposes. To diagnose HPV infections, 3 modalities can be used: (i) Pap smears for identifying cytological changes secondary to cervical infections; (ii) HPV DNA identification systems; and (iii) HPV serological tests.

Pap smears have been the 'gold standard' for the detection of HPV-related changes in cervical cells that can lead to cervical neoplasia. Routine Pap smear screening has been stunningly successful. It has decreased the rate of cervical cancer by 70%. Recent guidelines have been promulgated to guide the interpretation of Pap smears and their use in the management of cervical dysplasia.[17,18]

Several different types of nucleic acid identification techniques are used to detect HPV DNA. Only one test is currently commercially available, the Hybrid Capture II assay (Digene, Inc., Gaithersburg, MD, USA). This assay uses synthetic DNA probes in solution to detect HPV DNA in specimens. The test provides two different assay 'cocktails' to detect groups of 13 high-risk and 5 low-risk HPV types. It does not identify which specific HPV type is present. The assay gives a measure of viral load, identifying the amount of HPV DNA present.[19]

Polymerase chain reaction (PCR) provides a much more sensitive test for HPV. PCR-based tests can detect a broad spectrum of HPV types, and can distinguish between individual HPV types. PCR tests detect higher rates of infection than other DNA detection systems.[20] The assay's exquisite sensitivity can lead to false positive results. PCR tests that can identify individual virus types are frequently used in clinical and epidemiological research.[21]

Dot blot methods are inexpensive and relatively sensitive.[20] However, virus types that cause common skin warts may cross-hybridize with genital-type viruses. Weak signals may be hard to distinguish from false positives.[21] They are more useful in detecting actively replicating, productive infections rather than latent infections.[22] Dot blot methods are not useful for the clinical identification of wart virus.

In situ hybridization assays identify the wart virus within human tissues and, therefore, are useful in locating infected tissues. These assays are relatively insensitive, and will not detect latent infections.[21]

Southern blot assays using type-specific DNA probes remain the 'gold standard' for identifying and typing HPV in the research setting.[20] The technique is technically difficult and labour intensive. Southern blots are often used to confirm positive tests found by more sensitive methods such as PCR.[23] Table 3 compares the qualities of various methods for identifying HPV virus infections.[24]

IMMUNITY TO HPV INFECTIONS

HPV immunity has two components. Cell-mediated immunity is most significantly involved in resolving lesions. Immunosuppressed patients with decreased cell-mediated immunity often develop multiple, intractable warts, and are at increased risk of developing genital dysplasias and HPV-related anal and genital malignancies.[4] Regression of anogenital warts is accompanied by a localized increase in CD4 T-lymphocytes and macrophages.

The role of humoral immunity is less clear. Since HPV replicates in mature epithelial cells, it is most likely difficult for the immune system to have blood-born access to the virus. Of women with HPV DNA-associated genital lesions,

Table 3 Comparison of methods for diagnosing HPV infections[21,24]

Test	Sensitivity	Specificity	Advantages	Disadvantages
Visual inspection	Low	High	Easy to perform, rapid	Identifies only visible, proliferative lesions; cannot type HPV
Papanicolaou testing	Low	High	Inexpensive	Low sensitivity; cannot type HPV
Colposcopy	Moderate	Low	More sensitive than Pap testing	Low specificity; cannot type HPV
In situ hybridization	Moderate	High	Can localize HPV in tissue; good sensitivity and specificity	Time and labour intensive
Dot blot technique	Moderate	High	Easy to perform, rapid, relatively inexpensive; can type HPV	Less sensitive; cannot type HPV
Southern blot technique	High	High	Highly sensitive and specific; good ability to distinguish HPV types	Labour intensive, expensive, requires expertise; cannot localize DNA in tissues
Polymerase chain reaction	Very high	High	Extremely high sensitivity; good ability to distinguish HPV types	High risk of false positives; extreme care needed in handling of specimens
Solution hybridization	High	High	Relatively inexpensive; commercially available; identifies 'high risk' and 'low risk' HPV types	Cannot type individual HPV types; less sensitive than PCR

20–50% do not have detectable type-specific antibody.[25] The development of antibody to HPV types 6, 16 and 18 has been shown to occur an average of 11–12 months after infection. In a prospective study of previously uninfected young women, only 60% of the women seroconverted after infection with HPV.[26] Antibodies to HPV types 16 and 18 persisted, while HPV type 6 antibodies diminished over time. Humoral immunity is most likely 'type specific'. Antibodies to HPV type 16 have been shown to provide protective immunity against infection with other HPV type 16 variants.[27]

IS HPV A SEXUALLY TRANSMITTED DISEASE IN CHILDREN?

One of the difficult questions regarding genital and anal HPV infection in children is whether or not genital and anal warts are transmitted through sexual contact. Childhood sexual abuse has tremendous implications for the health of the child. Adults sexually abused as children have been shown to be at increased risk for mental illness, criminal behaviour, psychosomatic diseases, drug and alcohol abuse, welfare dependence, and a host of other negative and dysfunctional outcomes. Child sexual abuse is often very difficult to diagnose. Younger children may lack language skills to tell about their experiences. Older children may be hesitant to disclose because they have been threatened by the offender or fear reprisals. Many children perceive the abuse as their own fault. In some cases, the children feel a need to protect their abuser because their families are financially or emotionally dependent on him or her. The question remains as to how aggressively to pursue possible sexual abuse in children who present with anal and genital warts.

The question is further confused by the number of inconsistent studies in the medical literature. Many conclude that most anogenital HPV infections in children are sexually transmitted. Others reach the opposite conclusion. Studies have looked at different populations. Early studies used widely different methods of HPV detection and typing. Some laboratory methods used are subject to contamination or cross-reactivity with non-genital HPV types. Many of these methodologies were never tested in other laboratories. This lack of dependable methods may have led to inaccurate conclusions about HPV epidemiology.[28]

There are several arguments that have been presented that support the sexual versus the non-sexual transmission of anogenital HPV to children. These will be presented in counterpoint, first addressing the possibilities for non-sexual transmission.

Evidence that anogenital HPV infections are not likely to be sexually transmitted in children

1. Children contract the virus from their mothers during birth. The most compelling evidence in this regard is that infants are thought to contract juvenile laryngeal papillomatosis perinatally.[29] This disease is most commonly caused by HPV type 11, a genital-type virus. The disease most often initially presents during the first 2 years of life. Other studies have shown high levels of HPV in infants screened prospectively from birth for HPV colonization.[30] Whether these rates represent true colonization, transient colonization, or specimen contamination is unknown.

2. Children contract the virus from their mothers before birth. Rare cases have been reported of children being born with condylomata acuminata, suggesting vertical transmission.[31]

3. Children develop condylomatous lesions in the genitals and anus caused by common HPV types frequently found on the skin. Several authors have claimed that common, non-genital HPVs cause anogenital lesions in children.[32–34] These authors suggest that children commonly 'auto-infect' their ani and genitals from common skin warts, or that care-takers benign handling of the children and infants can lead to genital warts.

4. Genital-type viruses can infect the non-genital skin and, therefore, can be transmitted through routine, non-sexual physical contact. One study showed 27% of adult patients with genital or anal warts had the same type of virus isolated from their fingers.[35]

Evidence that anogenital HPV infections are often sexually transmitted in children, and that children are not likely to acquire genital-type viruses through non-sexual contact

1. Multiple studies of 'sexually non-experienced' adults have shown no evidence of genital or anal HPV infection and no evidence of HPV antibodies to genital-type viruses. In several of these studies, the women have been compared to sexually active women. Sexually non-experienced women are have not been found to be infected with genital HPV types.[36–41] Studies of HPV types 16, 18, or 6 seroconversion from negative to positive in college students show that the change occurs after the initiation of sexual activity.[40,41]

2. Studies of sexually abused and non-abused children show no evidence of anal or genital HPV infection in the non-abused children. McCann and co-workers found no genital or anal warts in children screened to determine they had not been sexually abused.[42] Gutman et al. studied 15 girls who had been sexually abused and 9 who were non-abused controls. Of the abused girls, 33% had genital-type HPV DNA isolated from cervical and vaginal specimens, and none of the controls were positive for HPV DNA.[13] One study of 11 girls with genital warts showed 10 to have specific evidence of abuse.[43]

3. Reported series of genital and anal warts in children consistently show a predominance of female children. Sexual abuse is known to occur more commonly to female children than to male children. Other sexually transmitted infections have been shown to occur more commonly in female children than in male children, in spite of the fact that STD in general are more common among men.[44] In series of anal and genital warts in children, females invariably outnumber males, indicating sexual transmission is more likely than casual transmission.[45–47]

4. A large, prospective study of a cohort of infants born to women at high risk for HPV infection showed no persistent HPV infection of the children.[48] The children were followed for 2 years after birth using PCR to detect HPV DNA. Of the 235 enrolled women, 151 had live births available for study. Of the women, 51% had HPV DNA detected in vulvovaginal specimens, and 74% had historical, clinical, cytological or molecular evidence of HPV infection during pregnancy. None of the infants had genital-type HPV DNA identified. Eight infants were positive for unclassified HPV. The authors concluded that perinatal transmission of HPV rarely occurs.

In summary, the rates of genital-type HPV in non-abused, non-sexually active children have been reported to be so widely divergent (0–72%), the only conclusion that can be reached is that the data are uninterpretable.[38] In an excellent review of the literature on transmission of HPV to children, Gutman et al. noted that studies that did not describe in detail how sexual abuse was determined or ruled out were more likely to attribute genital and anal HPV infections to casual, non-sexual contact.[23] This points out the need for careful epidemiological studies of HPV transmission in children. Because of epidemiological methodologies used in past studies combined with the problem of inaccurate laboratory tests having been employed, the final answer to the question of how frequently HPV is sexually transmitted in children remains elusive. Given the risks of sexual abuse to the health of the child, it is reasonable to address the question of possible abuse in any child presenting with genital or anal warts.

MANAGEMENT OF GENITAL AND ANAL WARTS IN CHILDREN

None of the therapies approved for treatment of anogenital warts in adults have been thoroughly tested in children. Physicians empirically apply information on adult therapies when managing childhood anogenital warts. A few retrospective studies have been published reporting the outcome of some treatments in children.

Benign neglect

Allen and Siegfried reported that the rate of resolution of anogenital warts was no better in children receiving treatment that in those receiving no treatment.[49] In children who are treated and do not respond, most anogenital warts eventually regress after treatment is suspended. It is reasonable to avoid treatment and let the warts 'run their course', particularly in children who are asymptomatic and who have competent immune systems. Some parents and children find the presence of anogenital warts quite distressing, and the lesions in children of these families may require treatment to defuse their anxiety.

Patient-applied treatment

Several patient-applied treatments are recommended for adult patients. Podofilox (0.05% solution or gel) is the most commonly used. It is a purified antimitotic component of podophyllin resin. In one series, 15 of 17 children treated with podofilox gel experienced complete resolution of their warts.[50] The gel was applied with an increasing frequency from one application per week to twice a day for 3 days, followed by a 4 day break when no application occurred. Each week, one more application was added to the regimen. Eleven of 17 children reported localized irritation from the treatment.

Another potential topical treatment is imiquimod cream (5%). Imiquimod cream is an immune-modulator with anti-viral and anti-cancer properties. It stimulates local lymphocytic reaction and induces the production of cytokines and interferon-α. In adults, imiquimod cream is used once daily at bedtime, 3 times a week for up to 16 weeks.[51] One small series of children treated with this regimen led to regression of lesions in 75%, with minimal local side effects.[51]

Oral cimetidine has been used successfully in treating recalcitrant non-venereal warts in children and adults. The drug has immunomodulary properties, and minimal side-effects, although it is not approved for use in children. Successful treatment with cimetidine has been described in a small series of children, using 30 mg/kg/day administered in three divided doses for up to 3 months.[52]

Trichloroacetic acid and podophyllin resin (10–25%) are not acceptable for use in children under any circumstance.[53]

Health care provider-administered treatment

Cryotherapy with liquid nitrogen is commonly used to treat genital and anal warts. The effectiveness of the therapy depends on the amount of time the cold liquid is applied to the wart. In children, it is often not well tolerated because of pain and anxiety. Other topical therapies include trichloroacetic acid and podophyllin resin (10–25%). Both cause pain, and potentially can scar the skin. Preparations of podophyllin resin are very unstable, and some of the compound can be absorbed through the skin. These two chemicals are not useful options for use in children.[53]

Ablation of warts with carbon dioxide laser or by surgical removal require the child to be anaesthetized, adding to the potential risk of adverse outcome. Both can cause significant postoperative pain and possible scarring.[15] The risk of recurrence of the warts after treatment is high. Since less intrusive methods of treatment are available, these methods should be reserved for extreme cases.

A trial of 'benign neglect' coupled with excellent perineal hygiene is probably the most judicious initial treatment for most children with anogenital warts.

USE OF DNA VIRAL TYPING IN THE MANAGEMENT OF CHILDHOOD GENITAL AND ANAL WARTS

The long-term significance of early infection with HPV in the anus and genitals is unknown. Studies have identified 'high risk' types of HPV in vaginal and anal specimens obtained from abused girls.[14,54] It is not known if this puts children at increased risk of developing squamous cell dysplasias and cancers as adults. Younger age at first sexual intercourse has been shown to be an important risk factor for HPV-related cancers.[4,10]

In adolescent girls and adult women, the role of HPV DNA typing in identifying people at risk for development of cervical cancer is debated. Several trials are currently in progress to assess the usefulness of HPV DNA typing in managing patients with abnormal Pap smears and dysplasia.

Most external, visible genital and anal warts do not harbour 'high risk' virus types, but are more likely to be caused by types 6 and 11. No prospective studies have been done to determine the value of identifying HPV DNA from vaginal, anal, and cervical specimens from sexually abused children. One problem in recommending follow-up for positive specimens is the difficulty in getting families with HPV positive abused children to comply with frequent check-ups for vaginal and anal complaints.[55]

PREVENTION OF GENITAL AND ANAL WARTS

Consistent condom use has been shown to decrease the likelihood of acquiring genital and anal warts.[55] The rate of infection increases with an increasing number of life-time sexual partners. Educating adolescents about responsible sexuality could potentially decrease the risk of infection.

Currently, several vaccines are being developed for HPV. The vaccines have been developed using 'virus-like particles' prepared using recombinant DNA to produce a non-infective antigen. These vaccines are currently being tested on groups of sexually active young women to determine if they can decrease the incidence of anogenital HPV infections and cervical cancer.[56]

Key points for clinical practice

- Genital and anal warts are caused by human papillomavirus (HPV). Some types of HPV are known to be associated with the development of anal and genital squamous cell carcinomas.

- Genital and anal warts can have several different clinical appearances. The most common presentation is 'cauliflower warts' (condylomata accuminata). Most external genital and anal warts in children are not caused by oncogenic-type viruses.

- Subclinical or latent HPV infections can be present in tissues in the absence of recognizable clinical lesions.

- Several different methods exist to identify and type HPV DNA. The clinical usefulness of these methods outside of the research setting in diagnosing HPV infections in children has not been determined.

- Immunity to HPV infections is primarily cell-mediated, but humoral immunity also occurs.

- Whether or not anal and genital warts in children result from sexual contact is debated. Much of the literature is inconsistent, and laboratory methods used in early studies were often not reliable. While further research should be done, it is prudent to carefully evaluate any child who presents with anal or genital warts for possible sexual abuse.

- The initial treatment approach to genital and anal warts in immune-competent children should be 'benign neglect' because most infections will resolve spontaneously, even if left untreated. Other treatment options used in children include topical podofilox (0.05% gel or solution) and topical imiquimod cream (5%). Neither of these preparations are approved for use in children.

- Use of condoms and limiting the number of sexual contacts can help prevent anal and genital HPV infections in sexually active teenagers. HPV vaccines are being clinically tested to induce immunity with the hope of preventing warts and cervical cancer.

References

1. Cripe TP. Human papillomaviruses: pediatric perspectives on a family of multifaceted tumorigenic pathogens. *Pediatr Infect Dis J* 1990; **9**: 836–844.
2. Baker CC, Phelps WC, Lindgren V, Braun MJ, Gonda MK, Howley PM. Structural and transcriptional analysis of human papillomavirus type 16 sequences in cervical carcinoma cell lines. *J Virol* 1987; **61**: 962–971.

3. Lorincz HT, Reid R, Jenson AB, Greenberg MD, Lancaster W, Kurman RJ. Human papillomavirus infection of the cervix: relative risk associations of 15 common anogenital types. *Obstet Gynecol* 1992; **79**: 328–337.

4. Sonnex C. Human papillomavirus infection with particular reference to genital disease. *J Clin Pathol* 1998; **51**: 643–648.

5. Beutner KR, Reitano MV, Richwald GA, Wiley DJ. External genital warts: report of the American Medical Association Consensus Conference. AMA Expert Panel on External Genital Warts. *Clin Infect Dis* 1998; **27**: 796–806.

6. Weitzner JM, Fields KW, Robinson MJ. Pediatric Bowenoid papulosis: risks and management. *Pediatr Dermatol* 1989; **6**: 303–305.

7. Maddox P, Szarewski A, Dyson J, Cuzick J. Cytokeratin expression and acetowhite change in cervical epithelium. *J Clin Pathol* 1994; **47**: 15–17.

8. Barrasso R, De Brux J, Croissant O, Orth G. High prevalence of papillomavirus-associated penile intraepithelial neoplasia in sexual partners of women with cervical intraepithelial neoplasia. *N Engl J Med* 1987; **317**: 916–923.

9. Ferenczy A, Mitao M, Nagai N, Silverstein SJ, Crum CP. Latent papillomavirus and recurring genital warts. *N Engl J Med* 1985; **313**: 784–788.

10. Koutsky L. Epidemiology of genital human papillomavirus infection. *Am J Med* 1997; **102**: 3–8.

11. Mount SL, Papillo JL. A study of 10,296 pediatric and adolescent Papinicolaou smear diagnoses in northern New England. *Pediatrics* 1999; **103**: 539–545.

12. Mangan SA, Legano LA, Rosen CM *et al.* Increased prevalence of abnormal Papinicolaou smears in urban adolescents. *Arch Pediatr Adolesc Med* 1997; **151**: 481–484.

13. Gutman LT, St Claire KK, Herman-Giddens ME, Johnston WW, Phelps WC. Evaluation of sexually abused and nonabused young girls for intravaginal human papillomavirus infection. *Am J Dis Child* 1992; **146**: 694–699.

14. Gutman LT, St Claire KK, Everett VD *et al.* Cervical-vaginal and intraanal human papillomavirus infection of young girls with external genital warts. *J Infect Dis* 1994; **170**: 339–344.

15. Siegfried EC. Frasier LD. Anogenital warts in children. *Adv Dermatol* 1997; **12**: 141–166.

16. Kiviat NB, Koutsky LA, Paavonen JA *et al.* Prevalence of genital papillomavirus infection among women attending a college student health clinic or a sexually transmitted disease clinic. *J Infect Dis* 1989; **159**: 293–302.

17. Solomon D, Davey D, Kurman R *et al.* The 2001 Bethesda System. Terminology for reporting results of cervical cytology. *JAMA* 2002; **287**: 2114–2119.

18. Wright Jr TC, Cox JT, Massad LS, Twiggs LB, Winkinson EJ. 2001 consensus guidelines for the management of women with cervical cytological abnormalities. *JAMA* 2002; **287**: 2120–2129.

19. Davies P, Kornegay J, Iftner T. Current methods of testing for human papillomavirus. *Best Practice Res Clin Obstet Gynaecol* 2001; **15**: 677–700.

20. Bovicelli A, Bristow RE, Montz FJ. HPV testing: where are we now? *Anticancer Res* 2000; **20**: 4673–4680.

21. Trofatter KF. Diagnosis of human papillomavirus genital tract infection. *Am J Med* 1997; **102**: 21–27.

22. Kiviat NB, Critchlow CW, Holmes KK *et al.* Associate of anal dysplasia and human papillomavirus with immunosuppression and HIV infection among homosexual men. *AIDS* 1993; **7**: 43–49.

23. Gutman LT, Herman-Giddens ME, Phelps WC. Transmission of human genital papilloma-virus disease: comparison of data from adults and children. *Pediatrics* 1993; **91**: 31–38.

24. Johnson K, Canadian Task Force On Top Periodic Health Examination. Periodic health examination, 1995 update: 1. Screening for human papillomavirus infection in asymptomatic women. *Can Med Assoc J* 1995; **152**: 483–493.

25. Carter JJ, Koutsky LA, Wipf GC *et al.* Natural history of human papillomavirus type 16 antibodies among a cohort of university women. *J Infect Dis* 1996; **174**: 927–936.

26. Carter JJ, Koutsky LA, Hughes JP *et al.* Comparison of human papillomavirus types 16, 18, and 6 capsid antibody responses following incident infection. *J Infect Dis* 2000; **181**: 1911–1919.

27. Xi LF, Koutsky LA, Galloway DA *et al.* Genomic variation of human papillomavirus type 16 and risk for high grade cervical intraepithelial neoplasia. *J Natl Cancer Inst* 1997; **89**: 796–802.

28. Konya J, Dillner J. Immunity to oncogenic human papillomaviruses. *Adv Cancer Res* 2001; **82**: 205–238.

29. Smith EM, Johnson SR, Cripe TP. Perinatal vertical transmission of human papillomavirus and subsequent development of respiratory tract papillomatosis. *Ann Otol Rhinol Laryngol* 1991; **100**: 479–483.

30. Pakarian F, Kaye J, Cason J *et al.* Cancer associated with human papillomaviruses: perinatal transmission and persistence. *Br J Obstet Gynaecol* 1994; **101**: 514–517.

31. Tang C, Shermata DW, Wood C. Congenital condylomata acuminata. *Am J Obstet Gynecol* 1978; **131**: 912–913.

32. De Villiers EM. Importance of human papillomavirus DNA typing in the diagnosis of anogenital warts in children. *Arch Dermatol* 1995; **131**: 366–367.

33. Obalek S, Jablonska S, Orth G. Anogenital warts in children. *Clin Dermatol* 1997; **15**: 369–376.

34. Cohen BA, Honig P, Androphy E. Anogenital warts in children. Clinical and virologic evaluation for sexual abuse. *Arch Dermatol* 1990; **126**: 1575–1580.

35. Sonnex C, Straufs S, Gray JJ. Detection of human papillomavirus DNA on the fingers of patients with genital warts. *Sex Transm Infect* 1999; **75**: 317–319.

36. Van Doornum G, Prins M, Andersson-Ellström A, Dillner J. Immunoglobulin A, G, and M responses to L1 and L2 capsids of human papillomavirus types 6, 11, 16, 18, and 33 after newly acquired infection. *Sex Transm Infect* 1998; **74**: 354–360.

37. Andersson-Ellström A, Hagmar BM, Johansson B, Kalantari M, Warleby B, Forssman L. Human papillomavirus deoxyribonucleic acid in cervix only detected in girls after coitus. *Int J STD AIDS* 1996; **7**: 333–336.

38. Dillner J, Andersson-Ellström A, Hagmar B, Schiller J. High risk genital papillomavirus infections are not spread vertically. *Rev Med Virol* 1999; **9**: 23–29.

39. Bonnez W, Da Rin C, Rose RC *et al.* Use of human papillomavirus type 11 virions in an ELISA to detect specific antibodies in humans with condylomata accuminata. *J Gen Virol* 1991; **2**: 1343–1371.

40. Carter JJ, Wipf GC, Hagensee ME *et al.* Use of human papillomavirus type 6 capsids to detect antibodies in people with genital warts. *J Infect Dis* 1995; **172**: 11–18.

41. Carter JJ, Koutsky LA, Hughes JP *et al.* Comparison of human papillomavirus types 16, 18, and 6 capsid antibody responses following incident infection. *J Infect Dis* 2000; **181**: 1911–1919.

42. McCann J, Wells R, Simon M, Voris J. Genital findings in prepubertal girls selected for nonabuse: a descriptive study. *Pediatrics* 1990; **86**: 428–439.

43. Herman-Giddens ME, Gutman LT, Berson NL. Association of coexisting vaginal infections and multiple abusers in female children with genital warts. *Sex Transm Dis* 1988; **15**: 63–67.

44. Anonymous. Gonorrhea in children under 10 years of age in Canada in 1984. *Can Med Assoc J* 1984; **134**: 1275.

45. Padel AF, Venning VA, Evans MF, Quantrill AM, Fleming KA. Human papillomaviruses in anogenital warts in children: typing by *in situ* hybridisation. *BMJ* 1990; **300**: 1491–1494.

46. Boyd AS. Condylomata acuminata in the pediatric population. *Am J Dis Child* 1990; **144**: 817–824.

47. Obalek S, Jablonska S, Orth G. Anogenital warts in children. *Clin Dermatol* 1997; **15**: 369–376.

48. Watts DH, Koutsky LA, Holmes KK *et al.* Low risk of perinatal transmission of human papillomavirus: results from a prospective cohort study. *Am J Obstet Gynecol* 1998; **178**: 365–373.

49. Allen AL, Siegfried EC. The natural history of condyloma in children. *J Am Acad Dermatol* 1998; **39**: 951–955.

50. Moresi JM, Herbert CR, Cohen BA. Treatment of anogenital warts in children with topical 0.05% podofilox gel and 5% imiquimod cream. *Pediatr Dermatol* 2001; **18**: 448–450.

51. Centers for Disease Control and Prevention. Sexually transmitted diseases treatment guidelines 2002. *MMWR Morb Mortal Wkly Rev* 2002; **51**: 54.

52. Franco I. Oral cimetidine for the management of genital and perigenital warts in children. *J Urol* 2000; **164**: 1074–1075.

53. von Krogh G, Longstaff E. Podophyllin office therapy against condyloma should be abandoned. *Sex Transm Infect* 2001; **77**: 409–412.
54. Stevens-Simon C, Nelligan D, Breese P, Jenny C, Douglas Jr JM. The prevalence of genital human papillomavirus infections in abused and nonabused preadolescent girls. *Pediatrics* 2000; **106**: 645–649.
55. Wen LM, Estcourt CS, Simpson JM, Mindel A. Risk factors for the acquisition of genital warts: are condoms protective?. *Sex Transm Infect* 1999; **75**: 312–316.
56. Frazer IH. The role of vaccines in the control of STDs: HPV vaccines. *Genitourin Med* 1996; **72**: 398–403.
57. Mu XC, Tran TN, Dupree M, Carlson JA. Acquired vulvar lymphangioma mimicking genital warts. The case report and a review of the literature. *J Cutan Pathol* 1999; **26**: 150–154.
58. Handsfield HH. Clinical presentation and natural course of anogenital warts. *Am J Med* 1997; **102**: 16–20.
59. Obalek S. Jablonska S. Orth G. Anogenital warts in children. *Clin Dermatol* 1997; **15**: 369–376.
60. Amiry SA, Pride HB, Tyler WB. Perianal pseudoverrucose papules and nodules mimicking condylomata acuminata and child sexual abuse. *Cutis* 2001; **67**: 335–338.

Christine Léauté-Labrèze Alain Taïeb

10

Diagnosis and management of Stevens Johnson syndrome

In 1922, Stevens and Johnson described two children with a very severe condition associating continued fever, painful conjunctivitis, stomatitis and a generalised exanthema.[1] Stevens Johnson syndrome is usually preceded by prodromes, such as respiratory illness or unexplained hyperthermia. After 1–14 days, severe erosions of mucous membranes occur with extensive involvement of the lips and exudative and sometimes purulent conjunctivitis. The extent of skin eruption is variable. Purple macules evolve within hours to bullae and, in the case of extensive involvement, an overlap with toxic epidermal necrolysis is possible. The dramatic presentation of Stevens Johnson syndrome requires hospitalisation. Its outcome is potentially severe but, with adequate management, morbidity and sequelae are minor.

Stevens Johnson syndrome is a rare disease. In individuals under 20 years of age the incidence rate is estimated at 6–8 cases per million per year with a peak incidence in the second decade of life.[2-4] *Mycoplasma pneumoniae* infection and drug intake have been identified as major precipitating factors of Stevens Johnson syndrome;[5-10] however, the pathogenesis of the disease remains unknown.

CLINICAL FEATURES

PRODROME

In most cases, the prodrome consists of an upper respiratory illness with fever, malaise, cough, rhinitis and sore throat.[1,5-10]

Dr Christine Léauté-Labrèze
Praticien hospitalier

Professor Alain Taïeb (for correspondence)
Chef de service, Unité de Dermatologie Pédiatrique, Hôpital Pellegrin-Enfants, Place Amélie Raba-Leon, 33076 Bordeaux cedex, France
Fax: +33 5 56 79 59 87; E-mail: alain.taieb@chu-bordeaux.fr

SKIN INVOLVEMENT

After 1–14 days, skin eruption occurs abruptly, consisting of symmetrical purpuric macules which progress to blisters and areas of epidermal necrosis (Figs 1 & 2). Skin involvement may be limited to a few target-like lesions or it may be extensive. Some patients develop wide-spread macules, which rapidly enlarge and may become confluent leading to some overlapping of the clinical picture with toxic epidermal necrolysis.

MUCOSAL INVOLVEMENT

All children with Stevens Johnson syndrome have two or more mucosal sites involved. The lips present haemorrhagic crusts with desquamation and denudation of the mucosa (Fig. 3). A severe stomatitis is associated and usually the child is unable to eat or drink and is at risk for dehydratation. In addition, oesophageal involvement is often underestimated and may worsen dysphagia, leading to malnutrition.[11] In rare cases, gastrointestinal bleeding occurs.[6,11] Severe conjunctival involvement may occur, leading to purulent conjunctivitis with photophobia (Fig. 4). Pseudomembrane formation is possible and eyelids may appear adherent, necessitating meticulous daily eye care. Erosive and painful genital involvement may be observed, especially in girls (Fig. 5). Anal erosions are uncommon, as is nasal mucosal involvement.

OTHERS

The respiratory epithelium can be involved and, if pneumonia occurs, it may be difficult to distinguish an infectious process from sloughing of the

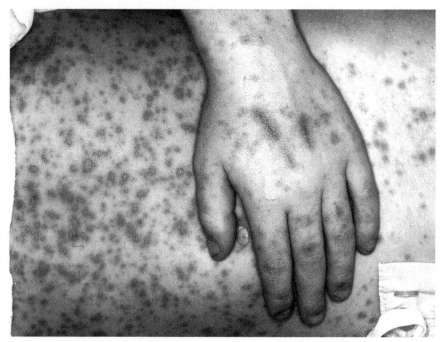

Fig. 1 Typical Stevens Johnson syndrome associating widespread blisters and areas of skin necrosis.

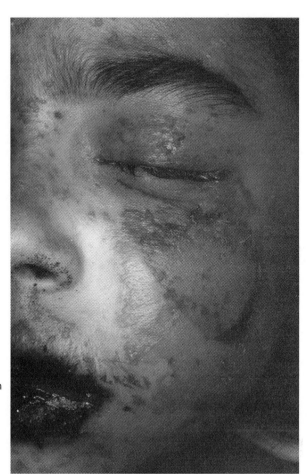

Fig. 2 Same patient as Fig. 1. Note TEN-like skin detachment on the cheeks and eyelids, in association with erosive cheilitis.

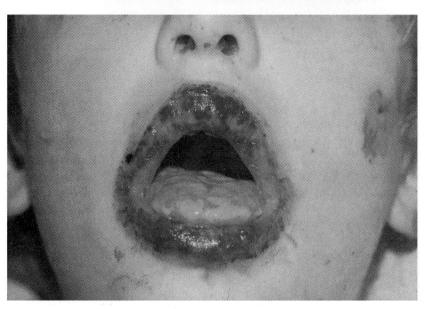

Fig. 3 Stevens Johnson syndrome. Erosive cheilitis and stomatitis.

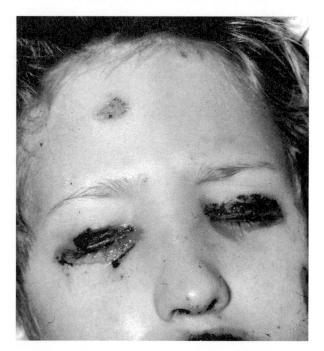

Fig. 4 Stevens Johnson syndrome. Conjunctival purulent discharge and photophobia.

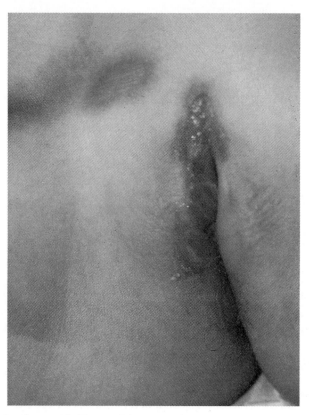

Fig. 5 Vulvar involvement in Stevens Johnson syndrome.

respiratory epithelium. Generalised lymphadenopathy is usually found, in association with spleen and liver enlargement. Arthralgias are sometimes found. Hepatitis is common, but myocarditis and nephritis are rare.

LABORATORY FINDINGS

A number of laboratory abnormalities may be observed, such as elevated CRP, leukocytosis and anaemia, but none are specific for Stevens Johnson syndrome. Fluid and electrolyte imbalance is common. Elevated liver enzymes are frequently found. Proteinuria and microscopic haematuria are rare.

PATHOLOGY

Skin biopsy is not necessary in most cases of Stevens Johnson syndrome. Pathological changes in the earliest skin lesion consist of accumulation of mononuclear cells around the superficial dermal blood vessels and epidermal damage which is the most characteristic feature, with keratinocyte necrosis leading to multilocular intra-epidermal blisters and extensive epithelial necrosis (Fig. 6). Epidermal necrosis results in incontinence of melanin pigment.

DIFFERENTIAL DIAGNOSIS

ERYTHEMA MULTIFORME

In the last 30 years, it has become widely accepted that erythema multiforme and Stevens Johnson syndrome, as well as toxic epidermal necrolysis, were all part of a single 'erythema multiforme spectrum'. Erythema multiforme was described by von Hebra in 1866[12] as an acute, self-limiting disease of the skin and mucous membranes characterized by symmetrically distributed skin lesions, located primarily on the extremities, and by a tendency for recurrence.[12-14] Indeed, there is little clinical resemblance between typical erythema multiforme and Stevens Johnson syndrome. In addition, aetiologies are different. *M. pneumoniae* infection and drugs are responsible for Stevens Johnson syndrome[5-10] whereas herpes virus is responsible for typical erythema multiforme.[13-19] The term erythema multiforme should be restricted to acrally distributed typical targets or raised oedematous papules (Figs 6, 7 & 8). Depending on the presence or absence of mucous membrane erosions, cases may be classified as erythema multiforme major or erythema multiforme minor.[15] However, although a consensus is easily obtained between experts in most cases of erythema multiforme minor, it is more difficult to reach in some cases of erythema multiforme major and Stevens Johnson syndrome, leading to confusion in the medical literature. Indeed, in every-day practice, children often present both typical and atypical targets more or less acrally distributed. Furthermore, a few patients have only mucous membrane involvement and are unclassifiable.[7] In both Stevens Johnson syndrome and erythema multiforme, an aetiological classification would probably be more satisfactory than a clinical classification based solely on skin eruption.

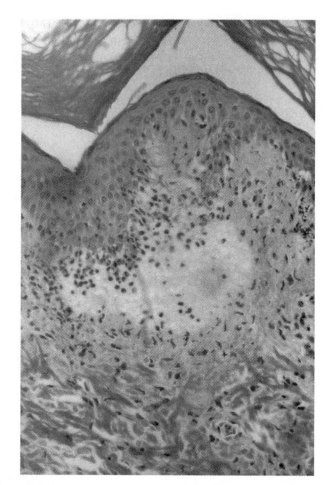

Fig. 6 Pathological changes consisting of keratinocyte necrosis, exocytosis of mononuclear cells, and oedema of the papillary dermis.

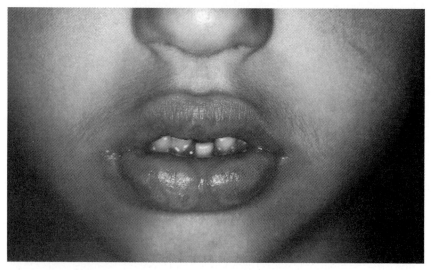

Fig. 7 Typical erythema multiforme with lip involvement.

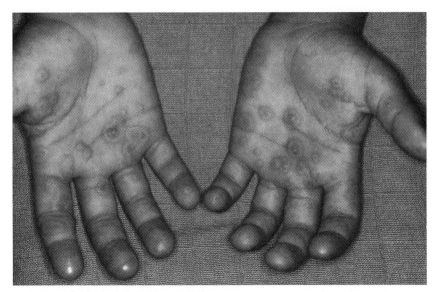

Fig. 8 Same patient as 7. Acral typical targets.

TOXIC EPIDERMAL NECROLYSIS

A similar debate concerns the overlap between Stevens Johnson syndrome and toxic epidermal necrolysis. Many arguments support the hypothesis that the two dermatoses are part of the same spectrum. The clinical presentations are very similar and the same drugs can induce both disorders.[20,21] Some authors propose the following categorisation: (i) Stevens Johnson syndrome for patients with widespread purpuric macules and a skin detachment of less than 10% of the body surface area; (ii) overlap Stevens Johnson syndrome/toxic epidermal necrolysis for patients with similar wide-spread eruption but 10–30% of skin detachment; and (iii) toxic epidermal necrolysis for patients with a skin detachment of more of 30%.[15] Childhood toxic epidermal necrolysis is mainly due to drugs,[20,21] and complications and sequelae are similar to those noted with Stevens Johnson syndrome but with greater frequency and severity.

OTHERS

Bullous drug eruptions can also mimic Stevens Johnson syndrome, but mucosal involvement is less common and the skin eruption is often polymorphic associated in the same patient with a maculo-papular rash, lesions affecting a pseudo-target pattern, and blisters.

Other differential diagnoses include Kawasaki syndrome when there is target pattern rash and major mucous membrane involvement, and auto-immune bullous disorders, which usually correspond to more chronic dermatoses.

AETIOLOGY

Identification of a single precipitating cause of Stevens Johnson syndrome is often difficult, and, although many precipitating factors (Table 1) have been implicated, *M. pneumoniae* and drugs predominate as major causative agents.[5–10]

Table 1 Precipitating factors of Stevens Johnson syndrome

Factors frequently involved in Stevens Johnson syndrome (more than 90% of cases)
- *Mycoplasma pneumoniae* infection
- Drugs

  Anticonvulsants – hydantoins, barbiturates, carbamazepine
  Antibiotics – sulphonamides, penicillins, tetracyclines
  NSAIDs – ibuprofen, naprosyn
  Anti-HIV drugs– nevirapine

Factors rarely involved in Stevens Johnson syndrome
- Immunizations – measles, hepatitis B
- Viral infections – enteroviruses, measles, HIV infection
- Bacterial infections – *Meningococcus, Streptococcus, Pneumococcus, Yersinia*
- Deep fungal infection
- Inflammatory bowel disease
- Cocaine
- Unknown cause!

MYCOPLASMA PNEUMONIAE

In our experience, childhood Stevens Johnson syndrome can be considered as an infection-driven disorder. Even though the aetiology remains unclear in some patients, in most, an infectious aetiology can be suspected on the grounds of various clinical, laboratory and radiological findings. *M. pneumoniae* infection is responsible for almost two-thirds of Stevens Johnson syndrome cases[7] – one-third of Stevens Johnson syndrome patients had proven *M. pneumoniae* infection, and in the other third *M. pneumoniae* infection was suspected because of pulmonary symptoms or upper respiratory tract manifestations.

DRUGS

A careful history taking of drug intake is recommended in cases of Stevens Johnson syndrome. However, a drug-induced eruption is not so frequent in our paediatric experience. Many children are given drugs at the onset of the disease, especially antibiotics. However, the causative role of the drug can not be proven in many cases.[22] The drugs commonly involved are anticonvulsants (barbiturates and hydantoins), non-steroidal anti-inflammatory drugs (ibuprofen), antibiotics (sulphonamides and penicillins) and more recently anti-HIV drugs (nevirapine). Cocaine-related Stevens Johnson syndrome should also be considered in adolescents.[23]

VIRUSES

Concerning viruses, herpes simplex infection is frequently incriminated in Stevens Johnson syndrome.[13–19] However, no case of typical Stevens Johnson syndrome has been attributed to herpes simplex.[9] The confusion rises from the difficulty in distinguishing erythema multiforme major from Stevens Johnson syndrome.[24] Stevens Johnson syndrome has been associated with other viral infections, such as measles[10] or HIV infection.[25]

IMMUNIZATIONS

Some rare cases have been associated with immunization[10,26] with living replicative viruses (measles) or viral antigens like those used for hepatitis B immunization. On rare occasions, bacterial infections (*Streptococcus, Pneumococcus*) or deep fungal infections have been implicated in Stevens Johnson syndrome.[10]

PATHOGENESIS

As previously mentioned, Stevens Johnson syndrome corresponds to a host-specific response to a wide variety of antigenic stimuli, but the pathogenesis remains unknown. The disease is characterised by a massive destruction of epithelial cells due to apoptosis. Cellular apoptosis is the consequence of increased levels of TNF-α and Fas-ligand in the early stage of the disease.[27] The mechanisms leading to the production of these cytokines is unclear, but it has been demonstrated that drugs can induce a specific CD4 or CD8 host-response suggesting an important role for a T cytotoxic response.[28]

MANAGEMENT AND COMPLICATIONS

Stevens Johnson syndrome has a protracted course of 4–6 weeks and is a potentially severe illness requiring hospitalisation in a specialised paediatric unit, but with adequate management, morbidity and sequelae are minor.

MANAGEMENT

Pharmacological investigation is recommended to eliminate a drug-induced Stevens Johnson syndrome, and, if an offending drug is suspected, it should be promptly withdrawn.[29] Careful symptomatic treatment (Table 2) is essential.[6,7,10,30] Nursing

---

Table 2 Symptomatic measures necessary in Stevens Johnson syndrome

Management at early stage (10–20 days)
- Hospitalisation in a specialised unit
- Withdrawing any offending drug
- No prophylactic antibiotics, only
    In case of pneumonia, antibiotics against *Mycoplasma pneumoniae*
    Prompt treatment of superinfection
- Daily skin care – signs of bacterial superinfection, use of antiseptic cares and non-adherent dressings, physical therapy to avoid contractures
- Daily mucous membrane examination and care – mucosal erosions and synechia, *etc.*
- Correction of fluid and/or electrolytic imbalance
- Caloric replacement: gastric tube?
- Analgesic measures – analgesia during skin care, topical xylocaine on stomatitis and genital erosions
- Intravenous immunoglobulins (no controlled studies)

Long-term follow-up
- Pharmacological investigations if an offending drug is suspected
- Ophthalmic follow-up
- Follow-up of genital sequelae (girls)

---

should include meticulous skin and mucous membrane care with daily ophthalmological examination. In the case of major mucous membrane and oesophageal involvement, intravenous fluids and nutritional support through a gastric tube may be needed.[11]

In childhood Stevens Johnson syndrome, prophylactic antibiotic treatment is not needed except in the case of an infectious background, when the probability of *M. pneumoniae* infection is high; in this case, the use of erythromycin is recommended.

The use of corticosteroids is controversial in Stevens Johnson syndrome.[31–33] In our experience, corticosteroids give no benefit in term of disease duration.[10] Nevertheless, some authors still recommend infusions of methylprednisolone in Stevens Johnson syndrome.[33]

Thalidomide has been proposed in severe Stevens Johnson syndrome or toxic epidermal necrolysis, but a detrimental effect has been found in patients with toxic epidermal necrolysis.[34] Recently, intravenous immunoglobulin therapy has been proposed in toxic epidermal necrolysis and Stevens Johnson syndrome, based on the inhibitory effect on Fas-mediated keratinocyte death by natural occurring Fas-blocking antibodies in human immunoglobulin preparations.[35] Encouraging open studies have been published.[36] However, these results need to be confirmed by larger, multicentre studies.

COMPLICATIONS

During the acute phase of the disease, superinfection, especially due to *Staphylococcus aureus* and *Escherichia coli* (urinary tract infections),[6,7] is frequent, requiring appropriate antibiotic treatment.

Ophthalmological complications include adherent pseudomembranes, corneal ulcerations, and later keratitis sicca, synechias and symblepharon.[6,7,10] Despite dramatic involvement of oral cavity associated with oesophageal desquamation, digestive sequelae are rare, but synechiae of the lips are possible. In young girls, chronic vulvovaginitis may occur leading to outbreaks of pain with dysuria and, in rare cases, vaginal or urethral stenosis as sequelae. Persistent skin changes are common including patches of hyper- or hypopigmentation. Shedding of the nails may result in transient anonychia in very severe disease overlapping toxic epidermal necrolysis.

In rare cases, Stevens Johnson syndrome may relapse, sometimes with mucous membrane involvement only.[10] In these recurrent forms of the disease, aetiology and pathophysiology remain unknown.

Key points for clinical practice

- Stevens Johnson syndrome is a rare disease with a peak incidence in the second decade of life.
- The pathogenesis of the disease remains unknown, but *Mycoplasma pneumoniae* infection and drug intake have been identified as major precipitating factors.
- Stevens Johnson syndrome should be differentiated from erythema multiforme which corresponds to a self-limited eruption with symmetrically distributed targets.

Key points for clinical practice (continued)

- Stevens Johnson syndrome is usually preceded by prodromes, such as respiratory illness or unexplained hyperthermia.

- All children with Stevens Johnson syndrome have two or more mucosal sites involved. The extent of skin eruption is variable, an overlap with toxic epidermal necrolysis is possible.

- Stevens Johnson syndrome has a protracted course of 4–6 weeks and is a potentially severe illness, but with adequate management, morbidity and sequelae are minor.

- If an offending drug is suspected, it should be promptly withdrawn to improve the course of the disease.

- Prophylactic antibiotic treatment is not needed, except in case of suspected *Mycoplasma pneumoniae* infection.

- Careful symptomatic treatment is essential.

- The use of corticosteroids is controversial in the management of Stevens Johnson syndrome, especially if an infectious aetiology is suspected.

- Intravenous immunoglobulin therapy has been proposed in toxic epidermal necrolysis and Stevens Johnson syndrome; however, efficacy needs to be confirmed by larger multicentre studies.

- Persistent skin changes are common including hyper- or hypopigmentation. Ophthalmological complications include adherent pseudomembranes, corneal ulcerations, and later keratitis sicca, synechias and symblepharon.

References

1. Stevens AM, Johnson FC. A new eruptive fever associated with stomatitis and ophthalmia. *Am J Dis Child* 1922; **24**: 526–533.
2. Chan HL, Stern RS, Arndt KA *et al*. The incidence of erythema multiforme, Stevens-Johnson syndrome, and toxic epidermal necrolysis. *Arch Dermatol* 1990; **126**: 43–47.
3. Storm BL, Carson JL, Halpern AC *et al*. A population-based study of Stevens-Johnson syndrome. *Arch Dermatol* 1991; **127**: 831–838.
4. Schopf E, Stuhmer A, Razny B, Victor N, Zentgraf R, Kapp JF. Toxic epidermal necrolysis and Stevens Johnson syndrome. An epidemiological study from West Germany. *Arch Dermatol* 1991; **127**: 839–842.
5. Sontheimer RD, Garibaldi RA, Krueger GG. Stevens-Johnson syndrome associated with *Mycoplasma pneumoniae* infections. *Arch Dermatol* 1978; **114**: 241–244.
6. Ginsburg M. Stevens-Johnson syndrome in children. *Pediatr Infect Dis* 1982; **1**: 155–158.
7. Prendiville S, Hebert A, Greenwald J, Esterly B. Management of Stevens-Johnson syndrome and toxic epidermal necrolysis in children. *J Pediatr* 1989; **115**: 881–887.
8. Assier H, Bastuji-Garin S, Revuz J, Roujeau JC. Erythema multiforme with mucous membrane involvement and Stevens-Johnson syndrome are clinically different disorders with distinct causes. *Arch Dermatol* 1995; **131**: 539–543.
9. Tay YK, Huff C, Weston WL. *Mycoplasma pneumoniae* infection is associated with Stevens-Johnson syndrome, not erythema multiforme (von Hebra). *J Am Acad Dermatol* 1996; **35**: 757–760.

10. Léauté-Labrèze C, Lamireau T, Chawki D, Maleville J, Taïeb A. Erythema multiforme and Stevens Johnson syndrome: diagnosis, etiology and management. *Arch Dis Child* 2000; **83**: 347–352.
11. Lamireau T, Léauté-Labrèze C, Le Bail B, Taïeb A. Oesophageal involvement in children with Stevens-Johnson's syndrome. *Endoscopy* 2001; **33**: 550–553.
12. von Hebra F. *Atlas der Hautkrankheiten. Kaiserliche Akademie der Wissenchaften*. Wien, 1866.
13. Huff JC, Weston WL, Tonnesen MG. Erythema multiforme: a critical review of characteristics, diagnostic criteria, and causes. *J Am Acad Dermatol* 1983; **8**: 763–775.
14. Howland WW, Golitz LE, Weston WL, Huff JC. Erythema multiforme: clinical, histopathologic, and immunologic study. *J Am Acad Dermatol* 1984; **10**: 438–446.
15. Bastuji-Garin S, Rzani B, Stern RS, Shear NH, Naldi L, Roujeau JC. Clinical classification of cases of toxic epidermal necrolysis, Stevens-Johnson syndrome, and erythema multiforme. *Arch Dermatol* 1993; **129**: 92–96.
16. Roujeau JC. What is going on in erythema multiforme? *Dermatology* 1994; **188**: 249–250.
17. Schofield JK, Tatnall FM, Leign IM. Recurrent erythema multiforme: clinical features and treatment in a large series of patients. *Br J Dermatol* 1993; **128**: 542–545.
18. Huff JC, Weston WL. Recurrent erythema multiforme. *Medicine* 1989; **68**: 133–140.
19. Brice SL, Krzemien D, Weston WL, Huff JC. Detection of herpes simplex virus DNA in cutaneous lesions of erythema multiforme. *J Invest Dermatol* 1989; **93**: 183–187.
20. Adzick NS, Kim SH, Bondoc CC, Quinby WC, Remensnyder JP. Management of toxic epidermal necrolysis in a pediatric burn center. *Am J Dis Child* 1985; **139**: 499–502.
21. Ringheanu M, Laude TA. Toxic epidermal necrolysis in children-an update. *Clin Pediatr (Phila)* 2000; **39**: 687–694.
22. Begaud B, Evreux JC, Jouglard J, Lagier G. Imputabilité des effets inattendus ou toxiques des médicaments. *Thérapie* 1989; **44**: 223–227.
23. Hofbauer GF, Burg G, Nestle FO. Cocaine-related Stevens-Johnson syndrome. *Dermatology* 2000; **201**: 258–260.
24. Weston WL, Morelli JG, Rogers M. Target lesions on the lips: childhood herpes simplex associated with erythema multiforme mimics Stevens-Johnson syndrome. *J Am Acad Dermatol* 1997; **37**: 848–850.
25. Mortier E, Zahar JR, Gros I *et al*. Primary infection with human immunodeficiency virus that presented as Stevens-Johnson syndrome. *Clin Infect Dis* 1994; **19**: 798.
26. Ball R, Ball LK, Wise RP, Braun MM, Beeler JA, Salive ME. Stevens-Johnson syndrome and toxic epidermal necrolysis after vaccination: reports to the vaccine adverse event reporting system. *Pediatr Infect Dis J* 2001; **20**: 219–223.
27. Paul C, Wolkenstein P, Adle H, Wechsler J, Revuz J, Roujeau JC. Apoptosis as a mechanism of keratinocyte death in toxic epidermal necrolysis and Stevens-Johnson syndrome. *Br J Dermatol* 1996; **134**: 710–714.
28. Mauri-Hellweg D, Bettens F, Mauri D, Brander C, Hunziker T, Pichler WJ. Activation of drug-specific CD4+ and CD8+ cells in individuals allergic to sulfonamides, phenytoin and carbamazepin. *J Immunol* 1995; **155**: 462–472.
29. Garcia-Dorval I, LeCleach L, Bocquet H, Otero XL, Roujeau JC. Toxic epidermal necrolysis and Stevens-Johnson syndrome: does early withdrawal of causative drugs decrease the risk of death? *Arch Dermatol* 2000; **136**: 323–327.
30. Barone CM, Bianchi MA, Lee B, Mitra A. Treatment of toxic epidermal necrolysis and Stevens-Johnson syndrome in children. *J Oral Maxillofac Surg* 1993; **51**: 264–268.
31. Rasmussen JE. Erythema multiforme in children. Response to treatment with systemic corticosteroids. *Br J Dermatol* 1976; **95**: 181–186.
32. Esterly NB. Corticosteroids for erythema multiforme? *Pediatr Dermatol* 1989; **6**: 229–250.
33. Kakourou T, Klontza D, Soteropoulou F, Kattamis C. Corticosteroid treatment of erythema multiforme major (Stevens-Johnson syndrome) in children. *Eur J Pediatr* 1997; **156**: 90–93.
34. Wolkenstein P, Latarjet J, Roujeau JC *et al*. Randomised comparison of thalidomide versus placebo in toxic epidermal necrolysis. *Lancet* 1998; **352**: 1586–1589.
35. Viard I, Wehrli P, Bullani R *et al*. Inhibition of toxic epidermal necrolysis by blockade of CD95 with human intravenous immunoglobulin. *Science* 1998; **282**: 490–493.
36. Morici MV, Galen WK, Shetty AK *et al*. Intravenous immunoglobulin therapy for children with Steven-Johnson syndrome. *J Rheumatol* 2000; **27**: 2494–2497.

A.Rashid Gatrad   Aziz Sheikh

11

Understanding Muslim customs: a practical guide for health professionals

THE MUSLIM NARRATIVE

CORE VALUES

Muslims follow the religion of Islam (Table 1) which traces its origins to the same Semitic soil that bore Judaism and Christianity. Its most profound tenet is a belief in Monotheism, summarised in the Declaration of Faith: 'There is no deity save God, and Muhammad is the Messenger of God'. Whispered almost universally by Muslims into the ear of their new-born or a dying loved one, the daily life and body of Muslim communities pivot around this very statement. Life's very purpose then is to realise the Divine, an aspiration that is achievable only through a conscious commitment to the teachings of Sacred Law.

Transmission and instruction in matters of Law was the role *par excellence* of the Emissaries of God, of whom Muhammad was but the last link in a chain that included such luminaries as Abraham, Moses, and Jesus of Nazareth. To Muhammad was revealed the Muslim Holy Book, *The Qur'an* – God's final communiqué with humanity.

SOURCES OF SACRED LAW

Sacred Law (*Shariah)* for Muslims is an all-embracing entity, dealing with every aspects of human existence and behaviour.

Dr A.R. Gatrad OBE PhD FRCP FRCPCH, Consultant Paediatrician, Manor Hospital; Senior Lecturer (Honorary), Birmingham University, and Honorary Assistant Professor, University of Kentucky, USA
Department of Paediatrics, Manor Hospital, Walsall NHS Trust, Moat Road, Walsall WS2 2PS, UK
Tel: +44 1922 656558; Fax: +44 1922 656742

Dr Aziz Sheikh BSc MSc MRCP MRCGP DCH DRCOG DFFP DipLSH&TM, NHS R&D National Primary Care Training Fellow
Department of Primary Care & General Practice, Imperial College of Science, Technology & Medicine, London, UK

Table 1 Salient features of Islam and Muslim society with glossary of Arabic terms

- Islam is an Arabic term which means 'peace' and 'submission to Divine decree'
- A Muslim is one who has submitted to God's ordinances and so is in a state 'of peace'
- Muslims follow the religion of Islam
- Over 1 billion Muslims world-wide, with Muslim majorities in almost 50 countries
- Muslims believe in Abraham, Moses, Jesus and many of the other Biblical prophets; Prophet Muhammad is God's final emissary
- The *Qur'an* is the holy book of Muslims
- *Sunnah* refers to the practices and sayings of Prophet Muhammad
- Sacred Law is derived from Revelation (the *Qur'an* and *Sunnah*) and scholastic human endeavour

- The *Qur'an* represents the primary source of Islamic Law
- The *Sunnah* (the words and practices of Prophet Muhammad) provides a second source
- *Ijtihad,* the process of deductive logic, represents the third main source, and it is this, which provides Sacred Law with its dynamism. Learned scholars (*Ulema*) are charged to respond to novel challenges that arise with technological advances by interpreting relevant verses from the Holy Qur'an and the practices of Prophet Muhammad and applying them to the problem in hand. Such deductions have a broad and clearly demarcated conceptual boundary; application is, however, almost always context specific.

In this paper, we describe and provide insight into Muslim customs that we believe are particularly important for Western-trained clinicians to be familiar with. Implicit in our approach is a recognition that, although the majority of these customs trace their origins to Sacred Law, factors other than religion have also proved important in shaping the practises of Muslim minority communities.

CULTURE, GENERALISATIONS AND STEREOTYPING

WHAT IS CULTURE?

Culture can be defined as the beliefs, values, and behavioural norms of a community; these are inherent features of a community and are, therefore, absorbed and acquired from the very first experiences in the world. 'The inherited lens through which we see, experience and interact with the world' is a metaphor commonly used by anthropologists and sociologists when seeking to explain the role of 'culture' in shaping outlooks – a role which is particularly important in determining notions of illness, disease, health and healing amongst

Table 2 Profile of world Muslim population

Name	Area (km²)	Population (million)	Muslims (%)
Afghanistan	652,225	25.8	99
Albania	28,750	3.5	70
Algeria	1,988,000	31.0	99
Azerbaijan	86,599	7.7	93
Bahrain	620	0.7	100
Bangladesh	147,570	128.1	88
Bosnia & Herzegovina	51,233	3.4	40
Brunei	5765	0.3	63
Burkina Faso	274,200	11.6	50
Chad	1,259,206	7.7	50
Comoros	2170	0.5	86
Cote d'Ivoire	322,000	14.0	60
Djibouti	22,000	0.6	94
Egypt	1,001,449	66.9	94
Eritrea	124,993	4.0	51
Ethiopia	1,153,000	62.1	50
The Gambia	10,380	1.3	90
Guinea	245,861	7.7	85
Guinea-Bissau	36,120	1.2	45
Indonesia	1,919,441	216.1	88
Iran	1,648,000	65.0	99
Iraq	434,923	22.5	97
Jordan	89,213	4.6	96
Kazakhstan	2,717,301	16.9	47
Kuwait	17,818	2.1	85
Kyrgyzstan	198,500	4.7	75
Lebanon	10,400	4.1	70
Libya	1,759,540	6.0	97
Malaysia	329,758	22.7	58
Maldives	298	0.3	100
Mali	1,239,999	11.8	90
Mauritania	1,030,701	2.6	100
Morocco	446,550	28.2	99
Niger	1,267,000	10.1	80
Nigeria	923,770	115.3	50
Oman	300,000	2.5	100
Pakistan	796,095	156.0	97
Palestinian Authority*	6220	2.7	85
Qatar	11,437	0.5	95
Saudi Arabia	2,253,300	20.9	100
Senegal	196,193	9.2	92
Sierra Leone	71,614	5.3	60
Somalia	637,638	10.7	100
Sudan	2,505,813	28.9	70
Syria	185,179	20.9	90
Tajikistan	143,100	6.2	85
Tunisia	162,155	9.5	98
Turkey	774,815	65.9	100
Turkmenistan	488,101	4.8	89
United Arab Emirates	83,600	2.9	96
Uzbekistan	447,399	24.4	88
Western Sahara	266,000	0.2	100
Yemen	527,969	16.9	100

Population figures and the proportion of Muslims are approximate.
*The territories of the Palestinian Authority (including the West Bank and the Gaza Strip) are still being negotiated with Israel.

Sources:
 The Observer (24 October 1999), London, UK, page 26 (World Extra).
 Population Reference Bureau, 1999.
 Figures supplied by the London embassies of most of the above countries in the year 2000.
 The World Factbook 1999, CIA.

Muslim communities. When discussing culture, it is important to recognise that culture is a dynamic entity; migration often accelerates the process of change, typically through the phenomenon of acculturation – the process by which minority cultures take on the features of the majority.

It is well recognised that religion-based cultures are typically slowest to adapt. The strong cohesive effect of a common religious tradition is perhaps not surprising (the Latin term *religio* after all means 'to bind') since the practises typically stem from a shared set of beliefs and are thus intricately interwoven into the very fabric of society.

CULTURAL COMPETENCY INITIATIVES

Qureshi and others[1] exhort that health professionals should have a comprehensive understanding of minority cultural traditions, whereas Kai[2] has argued that Britain is now too pluralist for this to be a realistic proposition; instead, professionals should be encouraged to value diversity through a commitment to practise and deliver patient-centred care. A third possible approach, and one that we favour, is that professionals be taught to understand the underlying narrative that acts as a cohesive force in shaping culture.

MUSLIMS WORLD-WIDE

There are in the world today an estimated 1.2 billion Muslims (Table 2).

Muslims in Britain

The British Muslim population is currently estimated at about 2 million (Table 3). Most have been economic migrants coming from south Asia; more recently, migration has continued for political reasons, drawing families from the Balkans, central and western Africa, and Afghanistan.

Muslims in the US

Approximately half (3 million) of the US Muslim population is comprised of indigenous first-generation converts; the remainder trace their origins, in the main, from the continents of Asia and Africa.[3]

Table 3 Ethnic breakdown of UK Muslim population 1991

Country/region of origin	Numbers (thousands)
Pakistan/Bangladeshi/India	774
Other Asians	80
'Other other'	29
Turkish Cypriots	45
Other Muslim countries	367
African Muslims (New Commonwealth)	115
Total	1410

FAMILY: THE BUILDING BLOCK OF SOCIETY

MARRIAGE – THE BASIS OF FAMILY LIFE

The *Qur'an* uses the simile of 'a garment' to describe the relationship that should exist between a couple: just as the role of a garment is to conceal blemishes, provide warmth, protection, and to beautify, so too must each of the pair strive to complement and enhance one another. In contrast, relationships that remain untied by the secure bond of matrimony are viewed as unstable and hence not conducive to the development of a wholesome society.[4]

Marriage is commonly seen as a union between two families. Parents of the prospective bride and groom will thus take into account a range of factors that include educational, ethnic, linguistic and family backgrounds when attempting to arrange marriage. Although free consent of bride and groom are an essential prerequisite to a valid union, parental coercion is sometimes present.

EXTENDED AND NUCLEAR FAMILIES

An extended family structure is typical of Asian and African Muslim families. It is important to realise that family dynamics in these cultures may be very different from those customary amongst people from the West. For example, amongst Asian people the family is more typically hierarchical and patriarchal when compared to European families. Males and females are encouraged to operate in different, yet complimentary, spheres of activity. For example, the male is typically seen as the bread-winner, whereas females are more concerned with domestic responsibilities. These generalisations should not, however, lead to stereotyping, as many Asian families are currently moving towards a nuclear family structure.

As a result of cultural adaptation, traditional family values are gradually being eroded with important ramifications. The breakdown of extended family units has resulted in changes in health-seeking behaviour, for example, with more young mothers now seeking advice on breast-feeding, behavioural problems with their children, and problems with alcohol and drug abuse in adolescents. Broken marriages, single parent families and increasing numbers of children born out of wedlock and 'put up' for adoption are some of the wider social effects that can, at least in part, be attributed to a disregard for the teachings of Sacred Law.

ANTENATAL CONSIDERATIONS

Recent developments in genetic and embryonic techniques have raised a number of ethical dilemmas concerning preconceptual issues. Summarised below are some of these that are of particular relevance when caring for Muslim patients.

GENETIC MANIPULATION, ASSISTED CONCEPTION AND ADOPTION

'Know your genealogy and respect your blood ties'[5]
Children have the right to be born through a valid union (marriage) and to know their parentage fully. Artificial insemination and *in vitro* fertilisation are, therefore, only licit if sperm from the spouse is used.

'We (God) created human beings in the most perfect form'[6]

Whilst genetic research and gene therapy may have positive uses in serving to restore health, care must be taken to ensure that other Islamic principles are not violated. An accurate and complete knowledge of one's pedigree is a fundamental right; only somatic cells (skin, for example) should be used in transplantation of genetic material, as hereditary characteristics are then not influenced. Conversely, germ cells (ovarian and testicular cells) carry important hereditary information and should, therefore, not be manipulated.

'Call the adoptive children by the names of their father'[7]

Adoption is generally frowned on in Muslim culture since the process involves the transfer of parental rights to the adoptive parents. Fostering is, however, encouraged instead, since no similar transfer of parentage occurs. In either case, the surname of the real father should be retained.

CONGENITAL DISORDERS

Genetic and non-genetic congenital disorders are more common amongst Britain's ethnic minorities. Choosing a partner from one's own ethnic group confers a significant risk (3–20%) of forming an 'at risk' couple, but the risk of these and other less common genetic disorders is substantially increased amongst cultures which sanction the forming of consanguineous relationships such as Pakistanis, Arabs and Turks. A study by Bundy et al.[8] has shown that offspring of such unions suffer significant more mortality and illness than other groups. Islam neither encourages nor discourages consanguineous marriages. Historically, the practice seems to have gained popularity as a means of safeguarding the family estate; the practice of endogamy, however, persists amongst minority communities largely because of difficulties in finding a suitable marriage partner from outside the family confines. Endogamy is marriage within a particular caste or clan known as biraderi amongst Asians. Muslims have long histories of intracommunity marriage and, as a result, have evolved separate and often unique gene pools.

PRENATAL DIAGNOSIS

Prenatal screening for haemoglobinopathies occurs in some parts of Britain, as the provision of such services is patchy. A new nationally linked antenatal and neonatal screening programme for thalassaemia and sickle cell disease is proposed in The NHS Plan.[9] Concern has recently been expressed regarding the higher than expected uptake of HIV screening amongst ethnic mothers, this possibly being the failure of antenatal staff to obtain informed consent from women who have difficulty in communicating in English.[10]

DELIBERATE TERMINATION OF PREGNANCY

'Each of you will have had his created existence brought together in his mother's womb, as a drop (nutfa) for forty days, then a leech like clot (alaqa) for the same period, then a piece of flesh (mughda) for the same period, after which God sends the angel to blow the spirit (ruh) into him'[11]

On the basis of this text, many Muslims conclude that a fetus acquires a soul at 120 days' post-conception – an important consideration in discussions regarding termination of pregnancy.[12,13] First trimester chorionic villous biopsy (*i.e.* performed before 120 days) and advances in therapeutic fetal medicine may in time lead to a greater willingness to engage in genetic counselling and prenatal screening.

'A mother should not be allowed to suffer on account of her child'[14]

An existing life, with its existing responsibilities and ties, takes preference over a developing one. If continuation of pregnancy places a mother's life in danger, then Muslim authorities agree that termination of pregnancy is justified. Termination for any other reason is strongly discouraged, particularly after 120 days of gestation.

THE ANTENATAL CLINIC

It is well recognised that infants born to Muslim mothers in the UK fare unfavourably when compared with the host Caucasian population. Possible reasons for this disturbing finding include poor attendance for antenatal care, socio-economic risk factors, and (indirect) racism. Difficulties in receiving care from female obstetricians, lack of privacy and communication problems are some of the explanatory variables that have been identified. A study by Watson[15] showed that the waiting times in antenatal clinics were the longest for Bangladeshis. They are the most recently arrived Muslim immigrants from South Asia and, therefore, least able to communicate in English.

The Asian Mother and Baby Campaign in the mid-1980s introduced the concept of 'link workers'. Their presence seeks to improve in-depth communication between the patient and the professional. One of the positive aspects of their work has been improved attendances at antenatal clinics by advising staff on relatively simple measures to ensure that procedures are culturally appropriate; a well-known example of such innovations has been the lengthening of hospital gowns[16] which cover most of the body and thus conform better with the Islamic code of modesty. Furthermore, it has been shown that where link workers were present there was a significant increase in birth weights of 'at risk' babies in Birmingham.[17] The increased proportion of female medical antenatal staff has further improved attendance.

BIRTH CUSTOMS

Familiarity with birth customs can help build confidence and rapport with parents – understanding the symbolism inherent in these rites also allows profound cultural insights.

THE PARENT–CHILD RELATIONSHIP

As has already been noted, children have a right to be born through a legitimate union with full knowledge of their parentage. The child also has the right to a good name, to be suckled, educated and, above all, reared in a stable, loving environment. In return, parents can expect to be treated with love and respect. And it is in recognition of this unique parent–child relationship that the noble Prophet reminded men and women of Faith that: 'paradise lies at the feet of your mother'.[18]

ADHAN

This means 'the call to prayer'. Within this call are incorporated the basic tenets of Islam: 'there is no deity other than Allah, and Muhammad is the Messenger of Allah' and concludes with a reminder that true happiness is dependant on the realisation of this truth. It is, therefore, only proper that the first word that a baby should hear is the name of his creator, Allah. These fundamental pronouncements serve as the pivot around which the life of a Muslim rotates, hence their symbolic significance at birth. The increased familiarity of the importance of this ceremony amongst British midwives and neonatal staff is very welcome.

TAHNEEK

This name is given to the Prophet Muhammad's practice of rubbing a small piece of softened date into the upper palate of a new-born infant. Where dates are not easily available, substitutes such as honey are used. A respected member of the family often performs this rite, in the hope that some of his or her positive qualities will be transmitted to the fledgling infant. The practise of only permitting access to partners into the delivery ward has its advantages, but may be seen by some as unduly restrictive, impeding the practice of this custom. Advice should be given against using honey as this can be a vehicle for infection with *Clostridium botulinum*.

TAWEEZ

This is a black string tied around a baby's wrist or neck with a pouch attached to it. It bears religious scriptures and should be handled with respect. It is believed by some that *taweez* will help protect the baby from illness and evil omens.

AQIQAH

A celebrity sacrifice of a sheep on the birth of a new-born baby is called *Aqiqah*. This is offered to Allah as a gratitude for every new-born child. It is usually performed on the seventh day after birth and the meat distributed amongst family members and the poor. Many will arrange for the sacrifice to be performed in their countries of origin, thus allowing the meat to be distributed where there is greater need, whilst simultaneously enabling disparate family members to partake in the celebrations.

NAMING SYSTEMS

The choice of a good name is a basic childhood right. It is hoped that the name will both inspire self-respect and give the child something to aspire towards in

Table 4 Some female names and their meanings

Aminah	Trustworthy
Faridah	Unique
Fatimah	The Prophet's daughter
Nafisa	Precious
Rabiah	Garden
Salma	Peaceful

Table 5 Some male names and their meanings

Abdullah	Servant of Allah
Ahmed	Praiseworthy
Hamza	The Prophet's uncle
Musa	Moses
Sa'eed	Happy
Tahir	Pure

the years that lie ahead. (Tables 4 & 5). As members of the extended family are involved in choosing the name, it may take a few days before an infant is named. Muslim names are easily identifiable to the trained eye. For those less familiar with Arabic, title names can be very useful. Commonly used titles include Muhammad, Hussain, Abdul, Ali, and Ahmad for males; female names often have the prefix or suffix Bibi, Begum and Khatoon.

SHAVING SCALP HAIR

A new-born child is innocent and free from the internal failings that grip human-kind. The significance of the symbolic act of removing scalp hair is to protect the baby from these failings which include avarice, lust, envy, and pride, to mention but a few. Scalp hairs that grow during intra-uterine life are traditionally removed on the seventh day of life, and an equivalent weight in silver given in charity.

CIRCUMCISION

The performance of male circumcision is a *Sunnah,* that is a practice approved of by the Prophet Muhammad. The *Sunnah* represents an accepted basis for the derivation of Sacred Law and it is not, therefore, surprising that the overwhelming majority of Muslims respect this teaching and have their male offspring circumcised. An advantage of early circumcision is that the child is immediately able to identify with his culture, which gives him a sense of belonging. If hypospadias is noted, parents should be advised against this procedure until further surgical advice is sought as the foreskin may be needed for restorative surgery. Female genital mutilation is not a Muslim custom. It is thought to have existed before the advent of Islam over 1400 years ago; it is practised particularly in parts of North Africa and other parts of the world,[19] but is illegal in the UK.

BREAST-FEEDING

'For each time she puts the infant to the breast, God will grant her Divine reward'.[20] Sacred Law positively encourages breast-feeding; ideally this should continue for a period of 2 years.[21] Muslim etiquette demands that women should not expose certain bodily parts to anyone except their husbands. Milk production may be adversely affected if there is no privacy and she temporarily opts for bottle-feeding.

As Muslim mothers will also typically breast feed for longer – particularly the Bangladeshi[22] – this is possibly the leading cause of iron-deficiency anaemia in this group. It is possible that with the process of acculturation, the incidence and duration of breast-feeding will decline in these communities unless pro-active strategies are adopted to emphasise the benefits.

ATTENDANCE FOR POST-NATAL CHECK

South Asians commonly encourage nursing mothers to remain predominantly indoors until at least 6 weeks after delivery. A medical appointment for the baby may, therefore, not be kept. It is possible that this custom began in response to the threat posed by infectious disease in many parts of the Indian sub-continent. High calorific food is encouraged to restore strength and improve milk flow.

SOME ASPECTS OF CHILDHOOD

OUT-PATIENT ATTENDANCE

Better communication and understanding of religious customs may improve clinic attendance. A recent completed audit by Gatrad[23] has concluded that, in a paediatric out-patient clinic, the 'did not attend' rate was significantly reduced from 50% to 13% over a 3-year period after a complex intervention programme that took account of the fact that the highest 'did not attend' rates were in the fasting month of Ramadan ('did not attend' rate during the fasting month in 1995 was 80% compared with 13% in 1998).

SURMA

This is an eye cosmetic sometimes used in young children; it has a variable, but potentially high, lead content. The sale of *surma* in the UK is now illegal. The very effective way in which health professionals joined forces with ethnic media services and ethnic communities at large to highlight the possible dangers of *Surma* use, is an excellent model for further health promotional activities.

RELIGIOUS EDUCATION

After school hours and during holidays, children will often attend a *Madrassah*, which are religious classes, teaching Arabic and the meaning of the Holy *Qur'an*. Parents often also express the hope that their children will be imbued with a respect for the values and customs encouraged by their faith. Although almost all children will memorise some portion of the *Qur'an,* a small minority, as have hundreds of thousands of children before them, proceed to memorize the entire text (a remarkable feat when one considers that it is approximately equal to the New Testament in length). Such children are afforded considerable respect within the Muslim community because of the important role they play in safeguarding and preserving God's final revelation.

There is now an increasing trend towards faith-based schools in Britain and other Western countries. At present, there are an estimated 90 Muslim schools in Britain, although only four are state funded.

PERSONAL HYGIENE

TOILETING

In 20% of 240 Muslim homes visited in Walsall during paediatric domiciliary visits in 1988–1989, there were toilet pans that were low and flush with the floor – Asiatic toilets (Gatrad A.R., personal observation). One has to squat in order to use such toilet pans. It is, therefore, not easy to adjust from a squatting to a sitting position in hospital toilets. To ensure that clothes are not soiled for prayers, some males squat or sit down when passing urine. In addition to toilet paper, many Muslims use water after any toileting (*i.e.* after passing urine or defecation).[24] Nurses should be aware of this custom as they may see patients taking a bottle full of water to the toilet. All toileting is done with the left hand and water may often spill onto the floor and be thought to be urine.

EATING

It is encouraged that food be eaten with the right hand – although some will use cutlery, others prefer to imitate the Prophet Muhammad and eat with their hand.

Foods allowed
Pork and alcohol are absolutely forbidden. If medicines contain these products then they are allowed if there is no other equally effective alternative.

Halal (lawful) foods are similar, but not synonymous, with Kosher foods. Fish with scales, shrimps and herbivorous animals that have been slaughtered in a particular way with concomitant blessings from verses in religious scriptures are allowed.

ORAL HYGIENE

Islamic law encourages personal hygiene, including the need to maintain good oral health. In Prophetic times, the method employed was to use the wood from the *Salvadora persica* tree.[25] This practice still continues among devout Muslims. Of relevance here is that it is widely regarded as a sign of respect to offer one's tooth-stick to friends and relatives. This raises the possibility of blood-borne transfer of infection resulting from trauma, in a population that has an increased prevalence of gingival disease.[26]

Table 6 Key messages on Islamic celebrations and religious education

- As the Islamic calendar is lunar (255 days), the two celebrations called *Eid-ul-Fitr* (end of fasting month) and *Eid-ul-Adha* (celebrating the end of pilgrimage to Mecca) 'go backwards' by 10 days every year. These two festivals are separated by approximately 2 months and 10 days

- During the month of Ramadan, all Muslims above the age of 10 years observe fasting – that is not taking any food or water from dawn to dusk

- *Hajj* is the visit to Mecca in Saudi Arabia to perform Pilgrimage at least once in the life-time of a Muslim if finances permit. *Umra* is a lesser form of *Hajj* that can be performed at any time of the year

- Madrassah – place where young Muslim children learn to recite the *Qur'an* and its meaning

RELIGIOUS FESTIVALS

Muslims follow a lunar calendar (about 9–10 days shorter than the solar year). Therefore, all festivities, including the fasting month of Ramadan, will alter every year by approximately 10 days (Table 6).

FASTING

During the ninth month of the Islamic calendar, fasting is obligatory on all Muslims from the age of 10 years. No food or drink is taken from dawn to dusk. This could be for a period of 18 hours if the fasting month was to fall in summer months in the UK. There is no restriction to consuming lawful food and drink (*halal*) from dusk to dawn.

Although 'expecting' mothers are exempt from fasting, many still chose to fast, particularly during the first trimester. Interestingly, fasting has been shown not to affect the mean birth weight of babies at any stage of pregnancy.[27] As Muslim mothers rarely smoke, and for religious reasons strictly avoid alcohol, intra-uterine growth retardation is likely to be caused by reasons other than these.

EID

There are two festival days a year called *Eid-ul-Fitr* (at the end of the fasting month) and *Eid-ul-Adha* (celebrating the sacrifice of Abraham) separated by about 2 months and 10 days. When the new moon is sighted, *Eid-ul-Fitr* is confirmed to be on the following day – thus there is uncertainty about it until the evening before. More often than not, confirmation of the sighting of the moon comes from Saudi Arabia, Morocco or Pakistan. Long-term prediction of *Eid* day can be made within a 3-day accuracy. Difficulties always arise, as the day is not fixed until 12–36 h before the event. Parents or relatives may request that their children be discharged from the ward early, if possible, to celebrate these days. All children in some schools with a large Muslim population are given a 'day off'.

HAJJ AND *UMRA*

Hajj is at a specific time in the Islamic calendar whereas *Umra*, a lesser form of *Hajj*, can be performed at any time. *Eid-ul Adha* celebrations coincide with the end of pilgrimage *(Hajj)* to Mecca in Saudi Arabia. When most schools and businesses close down for Christmas and the New Year, a sizeable number of Muslims go to Mecca to perform *Umra*. Children often travel with them. Most adolescent boys and men return with their heads shaven after *Hajj* or *Umra*. We have already raised concerns of the possibility of blood-borne infection by the use of a 'common' razor for shaving.[28] The Prophet Muhammad likened those that successfully emerge from the standing on the desert plane of *Arafah* during the pilgrimage to Mecca, beseeching Allah's forgiveness for past excesses, as pure, 'like the day his mother gave him birth' – hence the removal of scalp hair again.

As *Hajj* and *Umra* cannot be performed during menstruation, adolescent girls may request from their general practitioner the contraceptive pill, to temporarily delay their period. Research has shown that during *Hajj* time, there is a high rate of failure to attend outpatients.[29]

Each year, the Saudi authorities issue visas to an estimated 40,000 UK pilgrims. Although *Hajj* takes place over a 5-day period, most travellers stay for about 15 days. Appropriate advice about vaccination, heat and food hygiene are important. Present recommendations for meningococcus vaccine are two doses of ACWYVax (3 months apart) with conjugate Men C vaccination, if not already immunised against this strain.[30] Since 1999, medical help is available through the British *Hajj* Consulate located in Mecca.

END OF LIFE ISSUES

CARE OF THE DYING

Life is seen as a sacred trust from Allah. Thus suicide and euthanasia are categorically forbidden.[31] Death is not a taboo subject in Muslim society and is an area one is encouraged to reflect upon frequently. This is a time when Muslims seek each other's forgiveness for excesses that may have been inadvertently committed; therefore, 50 visitors in the space of a day would not be unusual. Members of the immediate family will stay by the bedside gaining strength from reciting verses from the *Qur'an* – having a copy on the ward is a kindness.

STILL-BIRTHS AND NEONATAL DEATHS

Parents may wish to administer or spray holy water called *Zam Zam* to the dying/dead baby. This water is obtained from the wells of Mecca. Muslims are always buried and never cremated. Any non-viable fetal part including the placenta should be buried as the latter is also considered part of the human body and, therefore, deserves equal respect. All still-births are named and can be buried in non-consecrated grounds, such as a garden, although in the UK they are buried in a cemetery.

Ideally, the face of any Muslim, young or old, after death should be turned towards Mecca, that is south-eastwards in the UK. When a Muslim dies, the eyes and mouth should be closed and the limbs straightened. It is a religious requirement that the body be buried soon after death – this can be within hours of death.

POST-MORTEMS

'The breaking of a bone of the dead is equivalent to the breaking of a bone of one who is alive'.[32] Post-mortems are, therefore, not allowed unless the law of the country demands it. Research into the use of MRI scans instead of post-mortem examinations should be encouraged[33] to help avoid the distress often caused by this procedure.

ORGAN TRANSPLANTATION

'Whosoever gives life to a soul, it shall be as though he has given life to the whole of Humanity'.[34] The majority of Muslim scholars, particularly those from the Arab world, agree that organs transplantation should be encouraged – this being justified on the basis of the principle in Sacred Law that states that 'the needs of the living outweigh those of the dead'.[35]

Other Islamic scholars from Asia, however, believe that the body is a 'trust' and, therefore, as custodians of our bodies we do not have the right to donate any part of it. The illegal trafficking in organs has not helped the debate in favour of acceptance. An important *Fatwa* (legal ruling) from the UK-based Muslim Law (*Shariah*) Council in 1995 was strongly supportive of Muslims donating organs, and deserves wider circulation and debate.[36] It is our opinion that this ruling will have widespread appeal, particularly amongst second- and third-generation British Muslims.

STORAGE AND BURIAL

Purpose-built mosques have their own cold storage fridges. Before burial, the body is ceremonially washed and shrouded in simple white pieces of cloth. Male community members follow the procession to the graveyard where a special prayer is offered and the deceased finally laid to rest facing Mecca.

BEREAVEMENT

Mourning is usually for a period of 3 days during which time the mood is sombre and reflective; friends and relatives will typically spend much time during this period recounting positive experiences with the deceased extolling his/her virtues. The inevitable sense of loss that occurs at the time of death is tempered by the belief that any separation is temporary, re-unification coming in the life hereafter. This loss need not be a completely negative experience, as it represents an occasion to reflect on social and spiritual relationships, and indeed on the purpose of life itself.

Sabr is an Arabic word which may be translated as 'an unconditional contentment with the Divine decree'. *Sabr* is one of the ultimate spiritual heights to which a Muslim aspires. Relatives and community members will encourage the family to practice and develop such 'contentment' in this their 'hour of grief'. During the loss of a child, the family will be reminded that children are 'pure' and 'innocent' and, therefore, assured of paradise.

CONCLUSIONS

Respect for religion and customs of all faiths is important if health professionals are effectively to deliver care that is truly patient-centred. Our experiences suggest that there is a willingness to do so in many quarters of the National Health Service. We hope that by filling this cultural void, our contribution will serve as a small step towards improving understanding between different cultures.

Key points for clinical practice

- Artificial insemination and *in vitro* fertilisation not licit unless sperm is from spouse.
- Genetic manipulation should only involve somatic cells and not germ cells.
- Adopted children should retain the surname of the real father.
- As a fetus is thought to acquires a soul after 120 days of gestation, Muslims may accept termination before this period.
- *Adhan* – after birth, the baby is inducted into the religion by a respected person whispering the basic tenets of Islam: *'there is no deity other than Allah and Muhammad is his messenger'*.
- *Tahneek* is the name given to the rubbing of a date into the upper palate of the new-born.
- *Taweez* – a black string attached around the neck or wrist of a baby – contains religious words
- *Aqiqah* is the sacrifice of a sheep after the birth of each child – the meat distributed to the poor.
- Removal of scalp hair is thought to protect the baby from basic human failings.
- All Muslim males are circumcised soon after birth.
- Islam promotes breast-feeding for 2 years.
- *Zam Zam* is water from the wells of Mecca – applied or administered to the sick.
- Muslims are always buried and never cremated.
- *Sabr* refers to an unconditional contentment with Divine decree.
- Muslims believe in the hereafter.
- Islam does not allow post-mortems which need only be done if the law of the land demands it.
- Organ transplantation – this is still a controversial subject amongst Muslims. The Islamic scholars are beginning to advise positively about donating and receiving organs.
- Bereavement period – this is for 3 days.

References

1. Qureshi B. *Transcultural Medicine*. London: Kulwer, 1994; 214–215.
2. Kai J. (ed) *Valuing Diversity*. London: RCGP, 1999.
3. Kamyar MH, Roya P. Issues in Islamic biomedical ethics: a primer for paediatricians. *Paediatrics* 2001; **108**: 965–971.
4. Al-Qaradawi Y. *The Lawful and the Prohibited in Islam*. Indianapolis, IN: American Trust, 1960; 148–236.
5. Ben Hamida F. Islam and bioethics. In: European Network of Scientific Co-operation on Medicine and Human Rights. *The Human Rights, Ethical and Moral Dimensions of Health Care*. Strasbourg: Council of Europe, 1998; 84.
6. Ali YA. *The Meaning of the Glorious Qur'an 95:4*. Cairo: Dar-al Kitab, 1938 (Translation modified).
7. Ali YA. *The Meaning of the Glorious Qur'an 33:5*. Cairo: Dar-al Kitab, 1938 (Translation modified).
8. Bundey S, Alam H. A five year prospective study of health of children in different ethnic groups with particular reference to the effect of inbreeding. *Eur J Hum Genet* 1993; **1**: 206–219.
9. Department of Health. *The NHS Plan*. London: Stationary Office, 2000.
10. de Zuleta P, Sheikh A. Antenatal screening for HIV *J R Soc Med* 1999: **92**: 545.
11. Al-Haddad A. *The Lives of Man*. London: Quilliam, 1991; 16.
12. El-Hashemite N. The Islamic view in genetic preventative procedures. *Lancet* 1997; **350**: 223.
13. Salihu HM. Genetic counselling among Muslims: questions remain unanswered. *Lancet* 1997; **350**: 1035.
14. Al-Qaradawi Y. *The Lawful and the Prohibited in Islam*. Indianapolis, IN: American Trust, 1960: 202.
15. Watson E. Health of infants and use of health services by mothers of different ethnic groups in east London. *Community Med* 1984; **6**: 127–135.
16. Rocheron Y, Dickinson R. The Asian mother and baby campaign. *Health Educ J* 1990; **49**: 128–133.
17. Dance J. *A Social Intervention by Link Workers to Pakistani Women and Pregnancy Outcome*. Birmingham: East Birmingham Health Authority, 1987.
18. Kamyar MH, Roya P. Issues in Islamic biomedical ethics: a primer for paediatricians. *Paediatrics* 2001; **108**: 965–971.
19. Kamyar MH, Roya P. Issues in Islamic biomedical ethics: A primer for paediatricians. *Paediatrics* 2001; **108**: 965-971.
20. Amini I. *Ta'een-e-Tarbyat-Koodakan*. Tehran, Iran: Islamic Publishers; 1998.
21. Ali YA. *The Meaning of the Glorious Qur'an 2:33*. Cairo: Dar-al Kitab, 1938 (Translation modified).
22. Gatrad AR. *The Muslim in Hospital, School and the Community*. PhD thesis, University of Wolverhampton, 1994; 198.
23. Gatrad AR. A completed audit to reduce hospital out-patients non-attendance rates. *Arch Dis Child* 2000; **82**: 59–61.
24. Abdalati H. *Islam in Focus*. Indianapolis, IN: American Trust, 1975; 61.
25. Johnstone P. *Medicine of the Prophet*. Cambridge: The Islamic Text Society, 1998; 230–232.
26. Bedi R. Oral health. In: Rawaf S, Bahl V. (eds) *Assessing Health Needs of People from Minority Ethnic Groups*. London: Royal College of Physicians, 1998; 109–120.
27. Cross JH, Eminson J, Wharton BA. Ramadan and birth weight at full term in Asian Muslim pregnant women in Birmingham. *Arch Dis Child* 1990; **65**: 1053–1056.
28. Gatrad AR, Sheikh A. *Hajj* and the risk of blood borne infections. *Arch Dis Child* 2000; **8**: 375.
29. Gatrad AR. A completed audit to reduce hospital outpatients non attendance rates. *Arch Dis Child* 2000; **82**: 59–61.
30. Department of Health. *Health Information for Overseas Travel*. London: Department of Health, 2001; 31–32.
31. Sheik A. Death and dying – a Muslim perspective. *J R Soc Med* 1998; **91**: 138–140.
32. al-Asqalani AIH. *Bullughal-maram*. Riyadh: Dar-us Salam Publications, 1996; 199–200.
33. Bisset R. Magnetic resonance imaging may be an alternative to necropsy. *BMJ* 1998; **317**: 145.
34. Yurdakok M. Paediatric ethics in the Holy *Qur'an*. *Arch Dis Child* 2001; **85**: 79–81.
35. Boubaker D. Xenogreffe et bioetique Islamique. *Pathol Biol* 2000; **48**: 454–455.
36. Anon. The Muslim law (Shariah) Council and organ transplants. *Accid Emerg Nurs* 1996; **4**: 73–75.

Harish Vyas Jonathan H.C. Evans

12

Management of a potential organ donor

Organ transplantation transforms the outlook for children with end-stage diseases. The initiation of organ transplantation in the 1950s and the subsequent advancement in surgical and immunosuppressive techniques has led to a marked increase in successful organ grafting. There continues to be, however a major shortfall in the availability of organs for transplantation. This is particularly acute in paediatrics, where the difference between organ supply and organ demand continues to widen. The factors responsible for this shortage are many, but include family or cultural reasons, medical staff misunderstanding about contra-indications, and the problems of donor management. All families should be offered the opportunity of organ donation, regardless of their religious beliefs, as the decision is a very individual one The issue of organ retention in the UK has exacerbated this problem recently. With no foreseeable increase in the number of donors, it is necessary to maximise the collection of organs from the existing donor pool.

Most organs used in transplantation come from beating-heart donors who are clinically dead but whose vital functions are artificially maintained in intensive care units. These patients have suffered irreversible damage to the brain stem and would be unable to breathe on their own if the ventilators were to be disconnected. Following the diagnosis of brain stem death and the identification of a patient as a potential donor, it is vital that intensive medical care is continued. This will ensure that donor organs remain viable for transplantation and improve on the organ loss.

Dr Harish Vyas DM (Notts) FRCP FRCPCH (for correspondence)
Consultant in Paediatric Intensive Care and Respiratory Medicine, University Hospital, Queen's Medical Centre, Nottingham NG7 2UH, UK

Dr Jonathan H.C. Evans MB BS FRCP FRCPCH
Consultant Paediatric Nephrologist, City Hospital, Nottingham, UK

Table 1 Causes of death where organ donation is suitable and safe

- Head injury
- Spontaneous intracranial haemorrhage
- Acute ischaemia/hypoxia
- Metabolic encephalopathy
- Acute primary brain stem haemorrhage/infarct
- Low grade CNS malignancy*
- Treated meningitis and sepsis

*Pituitary adenoma, haemangioblastoma, benign meningioma, choroid plexus papilloma, craniopharyngioma.

IDENTIFICATION OF DONOR

Even before brain stem death has been formally diagnosed, the local transplant co-ordinator should be contacted and made aware of a possible donor as soon as possible. The suitability of the patient as a donor can then be discussed before approaching the family.

Cadaveric organ donations remain the most important source of grafts for all forms of transplantation and an understanding of brain stem death is central to this procedure. Brain stem should be differentiated from persistent vegetative state (PVS), where the entire cortex is destroyed but the brain stem continues to function. Apnoea may be a manifestation of intensive care neuropathy and myopathy and should be excluded. Absence of brain stem function is essential before organ donation is contemplated.

Within current UK law, there is currently no statutory definition of death although the following definition was recommended by the Working Party of The Royal College of Physicians on behalf of the Health Departments:[1] 'a permanent loss of capacity for consciousness, permanent inability to maintain spontaneous ventilation and permanent inability to maintain spontaneous heartbeat'.

Brain stem death, however, is defined as: 'a permanent loss of function of all neuronal structures in the brain stem such that there is irreversible loss of capacity for consciousness and breathing'.

CAUSES OF DEATH WHERE ORGAN DONATION IS APPROPRIATE

> However many ways there may be of being alive, it is certain that there
> are vastly more ways of being dead, or rather not alive.
>
> Richard Dawkins, *The Blind Watchmaker*

A list of causes of death where organ donation is likely to be possible is shown in Table 1. In general, potential donors with known malignancies are pre-cluded from organ donation. A rare exception is made for patients who die from primary central nervous system tumours, which are well differentiated, slow growing, and known not to spread outside the skull.[2] Donor organ acceptance, though, is always considered in the light of the urgency of the illness of the potential recipient.

Table 2 Circumstances where organ donation is contra-indicated

- Hepatitis B and C, human immunodeficiency virus, active cytomegalovirus disease
- Creutzfeld-Jakob disease
- Intravenous drug abuse
- Male sexuality with active AIDs
- Malignancy
- Recipients of human-derived pituitary hormones, human-derived gonadotrophins or human-derived dura mater
- Undiagnosed acute or progressive neurological disorder with or without dementia

Severe bacterial infections, even meningitis and sepsis, are not contra-indications for donation as long as the primary infection has been adequately treated.[3,4] This is not commonly recognised and organ donation request is not sought.

CIRCUMSTANCES WHERE ORGAN DONATION IS CONTRA-INDICATED

There has been a progressive expansion in the types of organs transplanted over the last two decades with a consequent change in the absolute contra-indications for suitability of organs (Table 2). Infections such as HIV, hepatitis B and C, and cytomegalovirus are absolute contra-indications for organ donation. Male homosexuality or intravenous drug usage are absolute exclusion for donation, but not encountered commonly in paediatric practice.

Recent concerns about transmission of Creutzfeld-Jakob disease (CJD) and other human transmissible spongiform encephalopathies has led to the following groups of patients being excluded from routine donation of organs, tissues and blood. CJD is being increasing found in younger patients and consequently there has been great concerns about children being donors. Patients with proven CJD or patients with clinically suspected CJD are, therefore, excluded from donation, as are patients where there is familial CJD. Undiagnosed dementing or neurological illness in the patient or the family precludes donation.

Donor-derived malignancy diagnosed in the recipient is exceptionally rare.[5,6] Audit of transplant records with data on thousands of patients show that only skin cancers and lymphomas occur at a higher frequency in transplant recipients than they do in the general population. Common cancers (*e.g.* lung and bowel) are no more frequent in the transplant population. Nevertheless, most malignancies except certain CNS tumours mentioned above and non-melanotic tumours are absolute contra-indications.

There are, however, contra-indications that are more organ specific, such as liver disease or end-stage heart disease, which would preclude those organs for donation. Disease affecting one organ, however, should not preclude other organs from being harvested. With increasing utilisation of tissues and organs from higher-risk donors, novel strategies will be needed to ensure the continued safe supply of organs. There will always be a need to balance donor organ quality and numbers with the urgency of recipients need.

Table 3 Conditions under which the diagnosis of brain stem death should be considered

Inclusion criteria	Exclusion criteria – must not suffer from
Have proven diagnosis of a structural condition that is known to cause a brain stem death (*e.g.* traumatic brain injury, haemorrhage)	Drug intoxication, including sedatives, narcotics, anticonvulsants and paralytics should be excluded
The condition should be irremediable as demonstrated by the clinical course over a period of time	Metabolic derangement such as diabetes insipidus and hypernatraemia are due to brain death and not due to primary condition
Be unresponsive to stimuli	Endocrine disorders
Be apnoeic and maintained on a ventilator	Hypothermia (core temperature of < 35°C)

CLINICAL DIAGNOSIS OF BRAIN DEATH

Brain stem death can only be diagnosed if the exclusion and inclusion criteria have been satisfied (Table 3) It is also vital that all the brain stem reflexes are absent and there is irreversible apnoea, and that these criteria have been independently confirmed. The diagnosis of brain stem death in infants under 2 months of age is generally regarded as insecure, but those over this age would follow the same criteria as adults. Non-breathing anencephalic infants may be suitable for organ donation although it has aroused an enormous amount of ethical discussions.[7]

DRUGS AND EVALUATION OF BRAIN DEATH

The toxic effects of drugs either self-administered or those dispensed in the intensive care unit must be excluded before considering brain death. Most centrally-acting drugs depress respiration making apnoea testing of brain stem function difficult. However, other aspects of brain stem function, such as pupillary responses, remain intact. Drug screening as well as quantitative measurements of blood drug levels can assist in interpretation of clinical state. In practice, therapeutic sedatives should be discontinued at least 12 h before performing the first brain stem test. Clinical diagnosis of brain death may still be allowed as long as the drug levels of these sedatives are below the therapeutic range. If in doubt, plasma estimation should be done.

BRAIN STEM TESTS

There are three major components in testing for brain stem death: (i) tests of brain stem reflexes; (ii) tests of irreversible apnoea; and (iii) re-tests by another physician (preferably independent) often, though not necessarily, after an interval.

Brain stem reflexes

Brain stem reflexes must all be absent as shown by the following:

- No oculocephalic reflex – (doll's eye movement)
- No pupillary reflex to light
- No blinking when the cornea is touched
- No cranial nerve motor response
- No vestibulo-cochlear responses – no eye movement when ears irrigated with ice cold water
- No gag or cough reflex elicited by tracheal suction

Irreversible apnoea

Irreversible apnoea can only be confirmed under the following conditions:

$$PaCO_2 > 5.3 \text{ kPa}$$

The patient is pre-oxygenated with 100% oxygen for a period of 5 min and is given 100% oxygen at 6 l/min via a tracheal catheter during the test so as to avoid further hypoxic brain insult. There must be no respiratory efforts over a 5-min period of continuous observations. The role of hypoxaemic drive in this situation is speculative.

Re-testing by an independent physician

Re-testing by another clinically independent physician must confirm the above observations. One doctor must be a consultant and the other must be at least 5 years post-registration, but neither can be a member of the transplant team. The timing of the interval between the tests depends on the clinical circumstances, but should allow adequate time for all the members of the medical and nursing staff to be re-assured of the diagnosis. The legal time of death is when the first test indicates brain stem death, but declared only after the confirmatory second test. The parents may want to be present at the time of the testing which could help them come to terms with futility of further intensive care.

In the UK, brain stem death is confirmed clinically; however, other investigations have been used to support the diagnosis. Magnetic resonance angiography is logistically difficult to perform in a patient who may be haemodynamically unstable; however, it may demonstrate arrest of blood flow in the carotid siphon. Similarly, cerebral angiography shows arrest of flow in carotid siphon. Radionuclide imaging may be used to demonstrate the absence of cerebral perfusion; however, it is less reliable for infratentorial structures. Transcranial Doppler has the advantage of being carried at the bed-side and, in experienced hands, will shows absent or reversed diastole flow. Brain stem auditory-evoked potential is a test that is not affected by sedatives, but remains invalid in the presence of pre-existing deafness, haemotympanum or petrous temporal bone fracture. Electroencephalography has been very well evaluated in this situation; high levels of artefactual electrical noise may make the reading of the findings difficult in the PICU environment. It does not measure brain stem function.

All these tests have their own disadvantages and none are essential to the concept of brain stem death. Many countries have their own clinical practices for diagnosing brain stem death and this may include requirement for instrumental tests in addition to clinical tests.

PHYSIOLOGY AROUND DEATH AND PRESERVATION OF ORGAN FUNCTION

The vast majority of kidneys and nearly all non-renal organs used for transplantation are harvested from cadaveric donors. This has been facilitated by the emergent technology in intensive care units that enables the maintenance of physiological homeostasis. Even with intensive care support, it is, however, only possible to maintain the brain-dead donor in a state of physiological stability for a short period of time. The recovery of viable organs for transplantation is dependent upon appropriate medical management both before and after death is declared. The pathophysiological changes induced in the potential donor by brain death soon defeat all the aggressive resuscitative measures taken by the intensivist. It is thus imperative to expedite the process of organ harvesting whilst continuing the intensive care.

Brain death produces a cascade of pathophysiological responses, which are uniformly harmful to all the transplantable organs. These responses include haemodynamic instability, respiratory failure, endocrine disturbances, and intractable hypothermia. Haematological changes are also commonly seen. We have a poor understanding of the majority of mechanisms involved in this.

Donor management involves intricate resuscitative effort to overcome these problems and maximise the potential viability of all organs. Once this process is in place, there is a balancing of the priorities for different organs, but the basic management goals are to achieve haemodynamic stability.

MANAGEMENT OF THE BRAIN-DEAD DONOR

MONITORING

Central venous pressure (CVP) line is essential to monitor the hydration status. Brain-dead patients will not become tachycardic in response to hypovolaemia, and thus fluid balance will require CVP monitoring and will require greater attention to fluid input and output. Radial artery line is essential for blood pressure and blood gas monitoring. Continuous pulse oximetry allows oxygenation to be assessed. Rectal or urinary bladder catheter temperature probes allow continuous monitoring. Bladder catheter is necessary to ensure that the urine output is at least 1 ml/kg body weight/h.

MANAGEMENT OF HAEMODYNAMIC INSTABILITY

Once brain death occurs, the changes in cardiovascular derangement is very much dependent on the antecedent ischaemia and intracranial hypertension. There is an initial exaggerated vagal activity producing bradycardia. As the brain stem function ceases, Cushing's response predominates producing a 'sympathetic storm' with a hyperdynamic state including tachycardia and hypertension. There then arises an imbalance between right and left heart function producing capillary leak and pulmonary oedema in the lungs. The massive afterload may produce myocardial ischaemia compromising the postoperative cardiac function of the transplant recipient. Further ischaemia of the brain stem and the spinal cord results in loss of sympathetic tone producing bradycardia and diminished myocardial contractility. Combinations of other factors produce hypotension.

Table 4 Causes of hypotension
Hypovolaemia
Inadequate fluid resuscitation
Continued bleeding
Fluid restriction employed for management of raised intracranial hypertension
Polyuria – either iatrogenic or due to diabetes insipidus
Ventricular dysfunction
Myocardial contusion
Acute electrolyte imbalance
Acute pulmonary hypertension
Endocrine and metabolic abnormalities
Anterior pituitary dysfunction
Adrenal insufficiency
Diabetes insipidus

Hypotension

Causes of hypotension are summarized in Table 4.

Fluid management. Aggressive fluid resuscitation is the mainstay of sustaining adequate systolic blood pressure. Bolus fluid should be administered and the maintenance fluid should be adjusted to a level in excess of hourly urine output. Maintain the CVP at 8–12 mmHg.

Inotropes and vasopressors. These should only be used after adequate rehydration has been carried out. Previous studies have shown detrimental effects of dopamine in early and late kidney graft survival.[8] In addition, increased mortality amongst heart transplant patients was shown to be associated with the use of dopamine in the donors.[9] Yet in another large study, administration of dopamine or adrenaline was not a significant risk factor for delayed early or late graft survival of kidneys.[10] In two studies, reduction in inotropic support was achieved by addition of antidiuretic hormone (ADH)[11,12] with preservation of myocardial function and perhaps beneficial effects on lungs as a result of reduced need of preload. However, endeavouring to maintain a fixed blood pressure is not justified as long as perfusion is maintained – urine output and blood lactates are good proxy markers. With our current state of understanding, inotropes will continue to be used, and should not preclude donor selection. Using the lowest dose of the least detrimental agent is the preferred approach, but this is not always possible. The goal is to achieve a normotensive, euvolaemic state.

Corticosteroids. Although there are no randomised controlled trials reporting the advantage of corticosteroids, some studies have shown their benefits.[13,14] In refractory hypotension, we continue to use corticosteroids empirically.

Thyroxine. Low T3 is found in brain-dead patients, although T4 and thyroid stimulating hormone continue to remain normal, a picture found in many sick intensive care patients. In two studies, hormonal supplements have improved haemodynamic stability and prolonged donor stabilisation.[15,16] However, two randomised controlled trials have not confirmed the above findings even in a subgroup with impaired left ventricular function.[17,18] We currently recommend the use of T3 in intractable hypotension when all other measures have failed.

Dysrhythmias

Atrial and ventricular arrhythmias occur frequently due to multiple aetiologies. Raised intracranial pressure alters brain stem function, which may lead to arrhythmias. Electrolyte imbalances such as hypokalaemia and hyperkalaemia, hypomagnesaemia, hypocalcaemia and hypophosphataemia are common. Myocardial ischaemia may occur as a result of contusion or coronary hypo-perfusion during the 'sympathetic storm' or as a result of hypovolaemia. Ino-tropic infusion may precipitate arrhythmias especially in the presence of ischaemia, higher doses being particularly pro-arrhythmic. Hypoxia and hypo-thermia are also contributory factors.

The most common disturbances seen terminally are bradyarrhythmias producing hypotension. Despite progressive failure of atrial and junctional pacemakers, ventricular escape rhythms are not seen. There is gradual slowing of the atrial mechanism followed by AV block or a gradually slowing junctional escape rhythm. Other terminal rhythms may be observed: atrial activity alone, slow junctional rhythm or sinus bradycardia or ventricular tachycardia (VT). A corrected prolonged QT interval may precede the development of VT. J waves may be seen in both normothermic and hypothermic patients.[19]

The management of arrhythmias revolves around immaculate supervision of electrolyte balance. Hypokalaemia should be treated with potassium infusion and insulin infusion should be commenced for acute hyperkalaemia. Other electrolyte abnormalities should be corrected. Hypothermia should be avoided by active warming using warm air blanket. Adjust ventilation to correct acidosis aiming to maintain the pH at 7.38–7.45. Respiratory alkalosis reduces arrhythmias especially ventricular fibrillation. Bradycardias only require treatment if they produce hypotension. However, when it happens, bradyarrhythmias are resistant to atropine and only respond to chrono-inotropes such as adrenaline. Occasionally, pacing may be required. A cardiac arrest should be managed as per appropriate arrest algorithm and does preclude subsequent organ donation if resuscitated. Occasionally, parents may not wish to continue with these procedures and their wishes need to be respected.

MANAGEMENT OF RESPIRATORY FAILURE

With brain stem death, there is marked reduction in the patient's oxygen consumption. Consequently, ventilatory requirements are often minimal. An increase in ventilatory requirement indicates fluid overload or onset of infection. The main goal is to maintain normal PaO_2 (9.3–13.3 kPa). The lowest inspired oxygen should be used to maintain normal PaO_2 and aiming to maintain oxygen saturations greater than 95%. Peak end expiratory pressures (PEEP) of less than 5 mmHg should be applied to minimise atelectasis.

Excessive PEEP may impair cardiac output and make the lungs unsuitable for donation. Regular physiotherapy with bagging, suctioning and postural drainage is also essential to prevent atelectasis and secondary chest infection. Nasogastric tube should be left on free drainage to prevent aspiration. Monitoring of mixed venous gases may help in evaluating tissue oxygenation.

MANAGEMENT OF ENDOCRINE PROBLEMS

Diabetes insipidus

The most important endocrine problem in the brain-dead donor is diabetes insipidus, which is most likely related to inadequate anti-diuretic hormone (ADH) production by the posterior pituitary gland. The approach to the management of diabetes insipidus is strongly determined by the fluid balance of the patient. The initial strategy is to replace fluid followed by hormonal substitution with desmopressin or ADH. Although one study[20] reported delayed graft function in kidneys from donors who had received desmopressin, another study indicated a better outcome from donors with diabetes insipidus who received desmopressin.[21] A large randomised controlled trial showed no detrimental effect of desmopressin on early or late kidney graft function.[22]

Once a diagnosis of diabetes insipidus has been made (Table 5), our current practice is firstly to ensure adequate fluid resuscitation and secondly to administer a continuous infusion of desmopressin. The infusion rate should be titrated to allow urine production of 1 ml/kg body weight/h. Serum and urine electrolytes need to be measured hourly until a steady state urine output is achieved, then every 4 h.

Hyperglycaemia

Mild-to-moderate hyperglycaemia is commonly seen soon after brain death, usually normalising after 24 h, and is often diagnostic.[23] Cortisol and catecholamines released at the time of 'sympathetic storm' counteract the effects of insulin leading to reduced glucose uptake. Within 24 h, spontaneous resolution of hyperglycaemia occurs precluding pancreatic failure as a cause. Infusion of inotropes may exacerbate this mechanism. The other mechanisms producing hyperglycaemia are reduced brain glucose metabolism and the infusion of large volumes of dextrose-containing fluids during resuscitation infusions.

The blood glucose levels dictate management of hyperglycaemia. Maintain the blood glucose level between 8–13 mmol/l. Reduce dextrose-containing intravenous fluids and commence insulin infusion if the levels of blood glucose remain persistently above 13 mmol/l.

Table 5 Diagnostic criteria for diabetes insipidus

Serum	Urine	CVP
Sodium > 150 mmol/l Osmolality > 305 mosmol/kg	Sodium < 40 mmol/l Specific gravity < 1.005 Osmolality < 250 mosmol/kg Urine output > 3 ml/kg body weight/h	< 4 mmHg

MANAGEMENT OF HYPOTHERMIA

The loss of thermoregulation following brain stem death renders the patient poikilothermic and hypothermia is universal. There is radiant and convective heat loss and, in addition, administration of large volumes of intravenous fluid at room temperature may contribute to rapid cooling of the patient. The consequences of hypothermia are severe. It contributes to cardiovascular instability, arrhythmias, and cold diuresis. It shifts the oxyhaemoglobin curve to the left decreasing oxygen delivery at the tissue level and contributes to organ deterioration. Coagulopathy occurs if the core temperature drops under 32°C.

Prevention of hypothermia is essential once brain stem death is confirmed. The patient is moved to a cubicle, firstly to allow the family privacy but also to permit the ambient temperature to be elevated. We routinely cover the patient, especially the extremities and the scalp, with aluminium foil to avoid convective heat losses. We also use warm air blanket, warm intravenous fluids. Warm gastric or bladder lavage has been recommended in refractory hypothermia of < 35°C.

MANAGEMENT OF HAEMATOLOGICAL DISTURBANCES

Anaemia and thrombocytopaenia may be present due to the on-going underlying processes such as bleeding or sepsis. Blood products are usually avoided to minimise sensitisation. Following brain death, a hypercoagulable state arises associated with release of large amounts of fibrinolytic agents (*e.g.* cerebral gangliosides) into the circulation. Fresh-frozen plasma and cryoprecipitate may be required to correct coagulopathy, with extra quantities being available for organ removal in operative theatre.

SCREENING OF THE POTENTIAL DONOR

Once brain stem death has been confirmed, laboratory evaluation of the potential donor continues with both general and organ-specific testing. The exact investigations carried out depend on the centre and the country (Table 6).

Table 6 A typical set of screening investigations in the potential donor
Basic laboratory values: full blood count, complete biochemical screen, liver and renal function tests

- ABO blood group typing
- HLA typing
- Microbiological studies including cultures of blood, sputum and sensitivities if positive culture results available
- Viral serology:
    HIV, Epstein-Barr virus (EBV), cytomegalovirus (CMV), human T-cell leukaemia virus type 1 (HTLV-1), hepatitis B and C, and CMV
- Urinalysis, culture, and sensitivities
- Venereal Disease Research Laboratory (VDRL) test

ORGAN SPECIFIC SCREENING ISSUES

Kidneys
Intrinsic renal disease and trauma are two contra-indications for donation. Size mismatch between donor and recipient is not a problem; indeed kidneys from young donors do less well primarily because of an increased risk of thrombosis, particularly when transplanted into small recipients. Because of this, in the UK most paediatric centres do not accept kidneys from donors less than 3 years of age, although some adult centres will transplant the two donor kidneys *en bloc*.

Heart
Currently, the selection criteria for potential heart donation in the UK are very stringent. There should be no family history of ischaemic heart disease and the donor should be under 50 years of age. A normal 12-lead ECG is prerequisite, although caution is required in interpretation because ST-segment changes and J waves are often found in brain-dead patients. There should be no prolonged asystole prior to donation and a minimal requirement of inotropes (usually < 20 mmmg/kg body weight/min). The donor should have good arterial gases.

Investigations prior to donation include, cardiology evaluation, ECG, chest X-ray, echocardiogram and cardiac catheterisation if the donor is older than 45 years. These criteria are justified as mortality has been found to be markedly increased in recipients of impaired hearts compared to who received undamaged heart.

Lungs
The grounds for exclusion are major lung contusion, persistent atelectasis, and pneumonia. In addition, patients with chronic lung disease either due to cigarette smoking or other causes (such as TB) rules out donation. In intensive care, excessive ventilatory pressures need to be avoided and PEEP maintained around 5 mmHg. The lowest inspired oxygen should be used to maintain a normal PaO_2 and oxygen saturations of greater than 95%. Fungal contamination of the respiratory tract increases morbidity and operative mortality. Operative bronchoscopy is carried out to delineate anatomy, perform broncho-alveolar lavage, and re-expand atelectatic lung segments.

Liver and pancreas
In a very large single-centre series,[24] overall survival was approximately 50% with up to 18 years of follow-up. Liver transplantation is now being performed earlier in the course of the disease with highest priority being given to those with acute and fulminant disease. The most common reason for liver transplantations in the childhood population is extrahepatic biliary atresia followed by metabolic disorders, and acute liver failure. Advanced cardiovascular disease or peritonitis remain relatively absolute contra-indications to organ donation.

Insulin-dependent diabetes is the main indication for pancreatic transplantation although the overall success rate is currently low. The safety of conventional treatment at present greatly outweighs its benefits.

Other organs

Cornea: The medical history of the donor is checked to exclude corneal scarring or topical infectious eye disease. An organ transplant recipient cannot be a corneal donor.

Skin: Skin banks are relatively new in the UK. Donated skin is used by burns and plastic surgeons to cover severe burns, small non-healing infected burns, and ulcers. Multiple blood transfusion or organ transplantation precludes donation. The other factors that rule out skin donation include severe skin disorders, long-term steroid therapy or tattoos.

Bone: Parents are concerned about mutilation following bone retrieval; however, reconstruction using replica bone makes the appearance normal. Bone banks can store material for many years.

Heart valve: Donation requires previously normal heart valves.

THE OVERALL APPROACH TO THE DONOR AND THEIR RELATIVES

NURSING CARE

It is essential to continue intensive nursing of the brain-dead patient prior to organ donation. The intensification of haemodynamic management, meticulous fluid management and frequent laboratory investigation will necessitate at least two nurses at the bedside. Frequent turning of the patient is necessary to aid ventilation, perfusion and prevent pressure sores. This is only carried out if the patient is haemodynamically stable. To preserve and protect corneas, lubrication of the eyes is necessary. There needs to be continued honest communication and support for the family and close liaison with the transplant co-ordinators.

APPROACH TO THE RELATIVES

Families and relatives rarely offer organs for donation spontaneously. The clinician in charge with the nurse who has looked after the patient and formed a close relationship with the family should approach the family on the matter of organ donation. It is important for the doctor and nurse to be experienced in this procedure to engender confidence and also a positive belief in the whole process of transplantation. Doubt on the part of the health professionals creates confusion and discontent within the family. There has been a recent recommendation in the UK for minimal requirements for training in consent for organ transplantation.[25]

There is never a good time to broach the grieving family on the subject of transplantation. A recent survey by the Paediatric Intensive Care Society demonstrated that there is no consistency between units or individuals about the timing of approaching families to discuss organ donation. The nurse looking after the child may be the best person to determine the optimal timing. It may be best to approach the family either between the two sets of tests or after brain stem death has been established and confirmed by the second physician. The consent for organ donation cannot be rushed and the family need to be given the opportunity to decide without feeling coerced. There will always be families who refuse transplantation and their wishes need to be respected without the clinician feeling a sense of failure.

Some parents, who initially may be reluctant for any further intervention, may agree to organ donation if they realise that a coroner's post mortem would have to be performed anyway. Parents not given the choice about donation may later wonder why, and feel resentful that they were not given the opportunity to help. Parents wishing to be with their child when the ventilation is discontinued may still be able to donate heart valves and corneas after death.

Occasionally, the parents offer organs but it is obvious that the patient is not a suitable donor. Their generosity needs be acknowledged and they must be given a full explanation of the reasons for refusal. After the family have in principle agreed to donation, the transplant co-ordinator could be brought in to explain the procedures and investigations that must be carried out. Once the family have had all their questions answered, a written consent can be obtained and they can specify which organs they may wish to donate. The coroner must be contacted to consent to organ donation if the circumstances require it and may send a pathologist to be present during organ harvest. The role of the co-ordinator is to perform two very important tasks: one is organ procurement, but an equally important function is to continue to provide support for the transplant recipients as well as the donor family. Keeping the donor family informed about the outcome is a very important part of coming to terms with the death of their child.

It is the co-ordinator who will gather all the necessary information about the donor and organise a retrieval team. Separate teams for heart, lung, and abdominal organs are involved and harmonization is vital to minimise the warm ischaemic time of removed organs. The donor organs are then sent to the designated locations for transplantation. The recipient operation often commences prior to the actual arrival of the organ at the recipient institution.

STRATEGY FOR INCREASING ORGAN PROCUREMENT IN THE UK

Since 1990, the number of transplantations has remained relatively static or even declined in some countries. Transplantation is exclusively dependent on the selflessness of others and many studies have shown that the great majority of people are in favour of organ donation. The number of people who either become donors or offer donation, however, remains low and so limits the service. Non-heart-beating donors can provide a few kidneys, but very few people will die in such circumstances that their organs can be harvested for donation purposes. Live donation, especially kidney or part of liver or lung, will be limited by the requirement of major surgery on a healthy person. Xenotransplantation remains a controversial issue. For the foreseeable future, the bulk of the organ requirement will have to come from heart-beating brain-dead organ donors.

To increase donation, an innovative strategy is required in the UK. Spain has been particularly successful, concentrating on the training and education of medical and nursing professionals who have the burden of responsibility of raising the question of donation with the families. They have felt that educational campaigns directed towards the general population were expensive and results questionable and presumed consent laws were not invoked. Transplant co-ordinators are located in all potential donor hospitals. This approach has increased organ donor rate from 14.3 per million population in 1989 up to around 35 per million population in 1999. There was increase in organ retrieval by 90% during the same period despite a dramatic decrease in deaths from road traffic accidents.

In the UK, a recent consultative document produced by the Department of Health[25] incorporates some of the lessons learnt from Spain.[26] It sets out plans for the development of 'UK Transplant' to co-ordinate and promote organ procurement throughout the National Health Service. It also recommends an action plan for wider training and education. In addition, there are plans for wider publicity campaigns with an assortment of commercial organisations. Increased provision of critical care will be required for this to be successful. A more comprehensive understanding of the subject by medical and nursing staff will improve the availability of donor organs and so improve the outlook for many patients and families.

Key points for clinical practice

- Organ transplantation transforms live of children with end-stage organ failure.

- There is a major shortfall in the availability of organs for transplantation.

- Brain stem death is defined as: 'a permanent loss of function of all neuronal structures in the brain stem such that there is irreversible loss of capacity for consciousness and breathing'.

- Brain stem death is a clinical diagnosis and requires two clinicians to confirm it.

- Donor identification should begin early; meningitis and sepsis are not contradictions to donation.

- Approaching donor family requires confidence and also a positive belief in the whole process of transplantation.

- Aggressive medical management of potential organ donor can increase the supply of organs from the existing pool.

- Haemodynamic stability should be maintained using the least amount of inotropes possible.

- Vasopressin is increasingly used to reduce the dosage of catecholamines.

- Maintaining normothermia reduces complications such as cardiovascular instability, arrhythmias, and cold diuresis.

- Continuous infusion of desmopressin is essential when diabetes insipidus develops.

> ## Key points for clinical practice (continued)
>
> • To increase donation, an innovative strategy is required in the UK concentrating on the training and education of medical and nursing professionals, who have the burden of responsibility of raising the question of donation with the families.

References

1. Department of Health. A Code of Practice for the Diagnosis of Brainstem Death. Including guidelines for the identification and management of potential organ and tissue donors. London: Department of Health, 1998 <http://www.doh.gov.uk/pdfs/brainstemdeath.pdf>.
2. Lutz-Dettinger N, de Jaeger A, Kerremans I. Care of the potential pediatric organ donor. Pediatr Clin North Am 2001; **48**: 715–749.
3. Lopez-Navidad A, Domingo P, Caballero F et al. Successful transplantation of organs retrieved from donors with bacterial meningitis. Transplantation 1997; **64**: 365–368.
4. Little DM, Farrell JG, Cunningham PM et al. Donor sepsis is not a contraindication to cadaveric donation. Q J Med 1997; **90**: 641–642.
5. Penn I. Occurrence of cancers in immunosuppressed organ transplant recipients. In: Terasaki P. (ed) Clinical Transplants 1990. Los Angeles, CA: UCLA Tissue Typing Laboratory, 1990; 53–62.
6. Penn I. Malignant melanoma in organ allograft recipients. *Transplantation* 1996; **61**: 274–278.
7. American Academy of Pediatrics. Infants with anencephaly as organ sources: ethical considerations (RE9253). *Pediatrics* 1992; **89**: 1116–1119.
8. Marshall R, Ahsan N, Dhillon S et al. Adverse effect of donor vasopressor support on immediate and one-year kidney allograft function. *Surgery* 1996; **120**: 663–665.
9. Wahlers T, Cremer J, Fieguth HG et al. Donor heart-related variables and early mortality after heart transplantation. *J Heart Lung Transplant* 1991; **10**: 22–27.
10. Koning OHJ, Ploeg RJ, Van Bockel JH et al. Risk factors for delayed graft function in cadaveric kidney transplantation. *Transplantation* 1997; **63**: 1620–1628.
11. Pennefather SH, Bullock RE, Mantle D et al. Use of low dose arginine vasopressin to support brain-dead organ donors. *Transplantation* 1995; **59**: 58–62.
12. Chen JM, Cullinane S, Spanier TB et al. Vasopressin deficiency and pressor hypersensitivity in hemodynamically unstable organ donors. *Circulation* 1999; **100 (Suppl 19)**: II244–II246.
13. Novitzky D, Cooper DKC, Reichart B. Hemodynamic and metabolic responses to hormonal therapy in brain-dead potential organ donors. *Transplantation* 1987; **43**: 852–854.
14. Follette DM, Rudich SM, Babcock WD. Improved oxygenation and increased lung donor recovery with high-dose steroid administration after brain death. *J Heart Lung Transplant* 1998; **17**: 423–429.
15. Salim A, Vassiliu P, Velmahos GC et al. The role of thyroid hormone administration in potential organ donors. *Arch Surg* 2001; **136**: 1377–1380.
16. Orlowski JP, Spees EK. Improved cardiac transplant survival with thyroxine treatment of hemodynamically unstable donors: 95.2% graft survival at 6 and 30 months. *Transplant Proc* 1993; **25**: 1535.
17. Goarin JP, Cohen S, Riou B et al. The effects of triiodothyronine on hemodynamic status and cardiac function in potential heart donors. *Anesth Analg* 1996; **83**: 41–47.
18. Mariot J, Jacob F, Voltz C et al. Value of hormonal treatment with triiodothyronine and cortisone in brain dead patients. *Ann Fr Anesth Reanim* 1991; **10**: 321–328.

19. Logigian EL, Ropper AH. Terminal electrocardiographic changes in brain-dead patients. *Neurology* 1985; **35**: 915–918.
20. Hirschl MM, Matzner MP, Huber WO *et al*. Effect of desmopressin substitution during organ procurement on early renal allograft function. *Nephrol Dial Transplant* 1996; **11**: 173–176.
21. Rabanal JM, Teja JL, Quesada A *et al*. Does diabetes insipidus in brain dead organ donors protect acute tubular necrosis in renal grafts? *Transplant Proc* 1993; **25**: 3143.
22. Guesde R, Barrou B, Leblanc I *et al*. Administration of desmopressin in brain-dead donors and renal function in kidney recipients. *Lancet* 1998; **352**: 1178–1181.
23. Staworn D, Lewison L, Marks J *et al*. Brain death in pediatric intensive care unit patients: incidence, primary diagnosis, and the clinical occurrence of Turner's triad. *Crit Care Med* 1994; **22**: 1301–1305.
24. Jain A, Reyes J, Kashyap R *et al*. Long-term survival after liver transplantation in 4,000 consecutive patients at a single center. *Ann Surg* 2000; **232**: 490–500.
25. Anon. *Organ and Tissue Transplantation: A Plan for the Future*. Draft consultation document for comment. <http://www.doh.gov.uk/organdonation/actionplan.pdf>.
26. Anon. *Organ Donation in Spain: The Spanish model*. <http://www.transweb.org/reference/journals/wtgf/sept97/world_spain.html>.

Helena A. Davies Vin Diwakar

13

Learning and staying up-to-date – advice for trainees and career paediatricians

The challenge of keeping up-to-date with advances in medicine has never been greater. The National Library of Medicine search service now has access to 11 million articles on Medline, from 4300 current medical journals <http://www.nlm.nih.gov/medlineplus/>. Medical resources on the Internet are expanding rapidly, and patients are increasingly questioning of their doctors. Optimal use of available time and resources to ensure maximal learning is essential so as to stay up-to-date and provide the best quality care for patients.

Every doctor needs to know how to learn and how to stay up-to-date effectively. While Continuing Professional Development (CPD) and Continuing Medical Education (CME) are terms which tend to be reserved for consultants (at least in the UK), in reality they extend across the whole continuum of medical education from medical student to career grade doctor. Madden and Mitchell define CPD as:

> 'the maintenance and enhancement of the knowledge, expertise and competence of the professional throughout their career, according to a plan formulated with regard to the needs of the professional, the employer and society'.[1]

The emphasis of the learning may change, but the basic aim of developing knowledge and skills in order to practice more effectively applies from the first day as a medical student right up to the day of retirement.

In this chapter, we aim to provide some practical advice on how paediatricians at all levels can optimise learning and place this advice within a theoretical and evidence-based context. Although learning is aimed at increasing knowledge and

Dr Helena A. Davies MBChB(Hons) MRCP(UK) FRCPCH, MD
Consultant in Medical Education, Postgraduate Medical Education Centre, F Floor, Stephenson Wing, Sheffield Children's Hospital, Western Bank, Sheffield S10 2TH, UK (for correspondence)
E-mail: h.davies@shef.ac.uk

Dr Vin Diwakar MBBS MRCP(UK) MRCPCH
Consultant Paediatrician, Birmingham Children's Hospital, Birmingham UK

modifying attitudes and skills, ultimately the aim of enhancing all of these is to improve our performance in practice. Evidence presented concentrates on the extent to which different learning methods actually improve quality of care. We begin by considering how we learn.

HOW DO WE LEARN?

A search for a single best way of learning is likely to be fruitless. Many innovations in education theory and practice have occurred in the past 10 years.[2] We each learn in different ways, and can change our style of learning depending upon what we are trying to learn.[3] In a study of 366 primary care doctors who identified active clinical problems in which they needed more knowledge or skill to solve, 55 different learning methods were selected.[4] The type of problem was the major determinant of the learning method chosen. The challenge is to plan medical learning so that it is centred on daily professional practice.

LEARNING THEORY

Many theories have been proposed to explain how we learn, often influenced by the prevailing thinking in psychology. An exhaustive review is not appropriate here. Nevertheless, an understanding of some of the fundamentals of adult learning theory provides insight into how to learn and helps explain why certain types of CPD are more effective than others. Learning theories most important in the context of medical education are outlined – behaviourist, cognitive, and action reflection theories being particularly relevant. A broad overview of adult learning theory is then provided.

Behaviourist theory
Behaviourist theory is based on the work of Pavlov, and proposes that learning is the modification of behaviour which arises from the application of specific stimuli through the provision of reinforcement. The learner is trying to obtain something they want (positive feedback) or avoid something they do not want (negative feedback). Behaviourist theory has been useful in understanding the importance of feedback, but in the past two decades support has grown for more sophisticated cognitive or adult learning theories.

Cognitive theory
Cognitive learning theory proposes that new information and experiences are built into pre-existing meaningful and systematic knowledge structures (schema), which are based on previous experience. Learning involves the processing of information through problem solving. Learning is enhanced by linking it with previous knowledge.[5] Trainers can do this by establishing what learners already know and introducing teaching with a simple framework of ideas which links what is already known with new information.

Action-reflection theories
Kolb suggested experience had to be the learner's own for effective learning to occur. He proposed the experiential learning cycle depicted in Figure 1.[6]

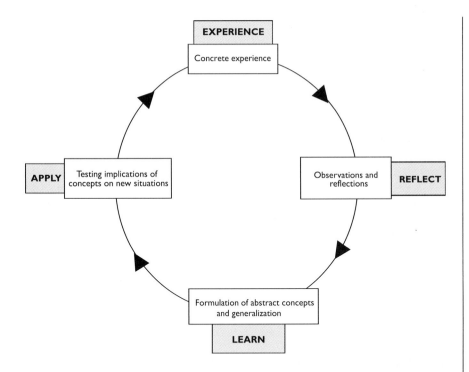

Fig. 1 An experiential learning cycle (Kolb and Fry).

Kolb proposed learners could, by reflecting on experience, gain theoretical understanding which, when applied to new situations, lead to new opportunities for experience and reflection. Kolb's theory is at odds with the traditional pattern of UK paediatric postgraduate education, in which theoretical knowledge is gained for the Part I MRCPCH examination; this may be taken after only 6 month's clinical paediatrics allowing little opportunity for improved theoretical understanding by reflection on experience.

Stanton and Grant[2] listed some important features for experiential learning: (i) commitment on the part of the learner; (ii) value placed on learner's experience; (iii) scope for independence in learning; and (iv) a structured basis to learning.

Schon proposed an even more advanced theory of professional development. He suggested that professional practice involves acting on the basis of intuition which is often unrecognised by the trainee.[7] Intuitive practice becomes clearer when trainees are allowed to reflect on their practice, yet junior trainees are usually taught in terms of clear-cut instructions which ignore the uncertainties of real-life medical decision making. According to Schon, learning is best achieved by reflecting effectively on practice.

Adult learning theory
Adult learning theory promotes the idea of independent learning. Knowles' adult learning theory proposes that learning must be relevant to the learner who must be able to relate the subject matter to what they do.[8] In medicine, a doctor's motivation to learn arises from clinical practice; but when trainees or

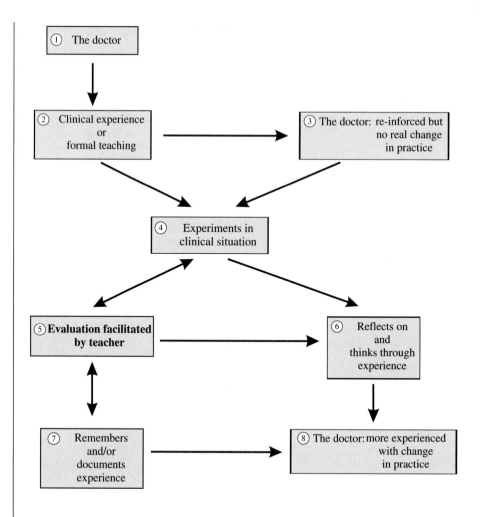

Fig. 2 A model of the learning process (*Adapted from*: Jarvis P. *Adult and Continuing Education*. London:Routledge, 1983: p70).

medical students learn, they must base it on their daily clinical experience. Knowles' theory gave rise to the modern concept of self-directed learning, where the learner takes control of the learning process and the teacher is more facilitator than provider of knowledge (Fig. 2).

Many of the themes which we have discussed are drawn together by Brookfield's principles of adult learning:[9]

• The learner's participation is voluntary

• Teacher and learner must have mutual respect for each other

• A spirit of collaboration must inform the learning process

• For doctors, clinical practice and reflection are a continuous process

- Critical reflection involves presenting the learner with alternatives which challenge the learner to seek evidence, ask questions and develop a critically aware frame of mind
- Adults need to be nurtured to develop self-directed learning skills.

DIFFERENT DOCTORS LEARN IN DIFFERENT WAYS

In the last 30 years, theories of how adults learn have become more and more sophisticated. Closely linked with adult learning theories is evidence that adults may learn in different styles.

The best known method of conceptualising and determining learning style is that of Honey and Mumford.[10] They provide a list of 80 self-assessment questions which take about 10 min to complete, and derive four basic learning styles:

1. **Activists**: learn best with new experiences, but bore easily. They like to be centre stage, to generate new ideas, to brainstorm and to have a go at anything.

2. **Reflectors**: learn best from activities in which they are allowed to stand back and think, to collect a lot of evidence and information before coming to a conclusion.

3. **Theorists**: like to adapt and integrate knowledge into logical structures, and learn best from activities in which models and pathways are provided to explain what is going on.

4. **Pragmatists**: like to try ideas out to see if they work in practice. They learn best when an explicit link exists between subject and job.

Most individuals possess a combination of all four styles in different proportions. Trainers should know what their learning style is so that they use methods appropriate to their own learning and to allow them insight if they have a trainee with a very different learning style. Course organisers should aim to provide a range of different learning activities to engage all the different styles of a learner.

Superficial and deep learning

Learners of any style may engage in surface (rote learning with little understanding) or deep (tries to understand what is learnt) learning. Deep learning is much more likely to be retained, but surface learning may get you through the exam next day! Deep approaches should be promoted, but changing trainees from a deep to superficial approach is much easier than *vice versa*. Marton showed that undergraduates with a deep approach changed to a surface approach when told that they would be tested on their factual knowledge, but did not change back to a deep approach when told that they would be tested for understanding.[11] Newble has suggested that traditional medical schools may not promote deep learning.[12] It is worth remembering that doctors who are completing their specialist registrar training and entering consultant practice at present were medical students at the time Newble and Marton were conducting their studies.

DOCTORS NEED TO BE MOTIVATED TO LEARN

Maslow suggested a hierarchy of learning needs, which must be satisfied before learning can occur at all.[13] The learner's physiological, physical, emotional and social needs must be met before higher order cognitive learning can take place. Stressed doctors working long hours with poor facilities for catering or accommodation are unlikely to learn. Similarly, teaching by humiliation is undesirable. Provision must be made for staff to deal with the stresses of everyday NHS clinical practice.

Motivation starts with the learner wanting to engage in learning. Two factors apply: (i) there must be some value to the learner; and (ii) the learner must expect to be able to do the learning task. Intrinsically, we may learn because we are interested in the subject itself. However, learners may also attach value to learning because of the outcome that it may bring: consultants see a reward in providing better care for their patients, young trainees are motivated more by the need to pass examinations (positive re-inforcement). Young trainees are also motivated by negative re-inforcement, the need to avoid failure. We can use the powerful motivating influence of assessment on trainees to ensure that we assess what is important for patient care, and not just what we find easy to test. Other motivating factors include the need to please people whose opinions are important to us and to compete against others and to achieve.

HOW DO WE KNOW WHAT TO LEARN?

In everyday practice, doctors use a range of informal means of determining what they need to learn.[14] Formal methods are used too, in formal appraisal and research. *The Good CPD Guide*[15] lists 46 such formal and informal sources under the following headings:

- Doctor's own experiences in patient care (*e.g.* difficulties arising in practice, knowledgeable parents, errors in practice, complaints, patient feedback, defining PUNS (patients unmet needs) and DENS (doctors educational needs)[16]

- Interactions with clinical team and department (*e.g.* clinical meetings, junior staff, changing job role, service development, organisational needs)

- Formal needs assessment (*e.g.* gap analysis, reflective practice, critical incident analysis, peer review, observation, practice review)

- Formal quality management and risk assessment (*e.g.* clinical governance)

- Peer review

- Teaching, research, lectures, reading journals.

Gap analysis
Actual performance is compared against a standard by self-assessment, peer review or objective testing.

Peer review

Doctors assess each other and make suggestions for appropriate education. Peer review varies in formality and may be internal or external. Other disciplines may be involved. Some researchers have achieved high levels of validity and reliability with formal methods of peer review although feasibility has been a difficult issue to resolve.[17]

Observation

A senior doctor, another professional or a patient observes the doctor performing a set task, formally or informally, and learning needs are identified.

Practice review

Review of formal documentation and prescribing, for example, can identify unmet learning needs.

Personal learning plans, reflective practice and educational supervision allow us to integrate our knowledge of learning theory, styles and motivation with analysis of learning needs.

PERSONAL LEARNING PLANS

Learning needs, once identified, are best used to inform a personal learning plan. The essential elements of the personal learning plan are to identify:

- What do you need to learn?

- Why do you need to learn it?

- How are you going to learn it?

- When are you going to learn it by?

- How will you know when you have learnt it?

- How does what you have learnt link with what you already know and what you need to learn in the future?[18]

Personal learning plans have a central role at all levels of medical education. They are consistent with theories of adult learning and have been used in a variety of settings including medicine. Learning contracts have been used effectively in the senior house officer grade.[19] Principals in general practice using portfolios based on personal learning plans covered a wider range of topics and learning activities when compared with a matched cohort undertaking 'traditional' continuing medical education activities.[20] The UK Department of Health now promotes the use of personal learning plans within its strategy for continuing professional development.[21]

Personal learning plans allow doctors to prioritise and justify areas for learning in the context of both individual and organisational objectives. Autonomy in choosing what, when, and how to learn is strengthened, not weakened, within an overall aim of improved patient care and better use of resources.[18] Many doctors are concerned that the art of medical practice is being swamped by political directives which assume that the only way to improve patient care is to be involved in a complex system of quality control.

In fact, professional practice is more holistic because it is unpredictable. Personal learning plans help us to analyse the complexity of professional practice in order to identify what is needed for improved patient care.

Educational supervision

Most doctors find self-directed learning challenging, and most examples of effective professional learning have identified the need for a facilitator. For career grade staff, this role may be taken by a peer at the same stage of professional development or by a non-medical professional. Nurses were using personal learning plans long before doctors and may have significant skills in facilitation. For trainees, facilitation usually falls to the educational supervisor.

Educational supervisors need to have a range of abilities. Wall[22] identified the main needs from an extensive literature search, analysis of the key themes in 11 'Teaching the Teachers' courses, and questionnaire survey of 593 consultants and doctors in training. These main needs were: (i) giving feedback constructively; (ii) building a good educational climate; (iii) assessing trainees' learning needs; (iv) keeping up-to-date as a teacher; and (v) assessing trainees. Training courses for educational supervisors should cover all of these areas, although further evaluation is needed to see whether such courses do improve the educational climate and lead to better patient care.

Reflective practice

The concept of reflective practice is built around the learning cycle. It is based on the premise that reflection on what has happened or been learned will improve retention of knowledge and increase the likelihood of change taking place. There are a number of practical applications of reflective practice that are useful and relevant to day-to-day continuing professional development. Portfolios and critical incident analysis are particularly good examples of how we can use the principles of reflective practice to enhance our own learning, (see below). The process of critically thinking about experiences encouraged by all forms of reflective practice is more likely to produce deep learning (as opposed to surface learning) than didactic teaching.

MAKING LEARNING EFFECTIVE – THE EVIDENCE

At postgraduate level, the key outcomes from CPD/CME/training should be improved professional practice and patient outcomes. There is now a considerable body of evidence on how this can be done most effectively.

FORMAL DIDACTIC CME IS NOT EFFECTIVE AT IMPROVING PRACTICE

The traditional format for consultant CME and for formal educational activities at all levels has been a didactic model, often centred around lectures. Increasingly, it is being recognised that learning is improved if principles of adult learning which encourage interaction, reflection, *etc.* are applied. A number of authors have examined the effectiveness of a range of CME strategies. Key themes which emerge include the relative ineffectiveness of traditional didactic lecture-based CME compared with strategies which are both more specifically tailored to an individual doctor's needs and more closely linked with practice.[23–25]

MAKING THE MOST OF FORMAL CME

Although didactic formal CME has been shown to be less effective than many other methods, it remains an important part of CPD for many doctors, both during training and once consultants. Some quite simple techniques can enhance learning from such activities. Importantly, simply writing down key learning points and/or possible areas for change within professional practice will improve the effectiveness of formal CME in modifying professional practice. Interestingly, it does not seem to make any difference whether or not the doctor signs up to this change or simply just records it.[26] Perhaps this is a reflection of the importance of intrinsic *versus* extrinsic motivation to change and learn.

SO WHAT IS EFFECTIVE CME/CPD?

In addition, there is some evidence that interactive CME sessions that encourage participant activity and provide an opportunity to practice practical skills are more effective than didactic lecture-based sessions in changing physician performance. In a review of controlled trials of formal didactic and/or interactive CME interventions, none of the identified purely didactic sessions had a discernible effect on physician performance while sessions that were interactive such as role-plays, case discussions and hands-on practice sessions generally had a positive effect on physician behaviour.[23] This review also suggested that sessions which were sequenced were more effective and postulated that the learn-work-learn opportunity provided by sequenced sessions allows learning to be translated into practice and then re-inforced at a further session. This fits well with the experiential learning cycle model described earlier. The most effective methods have in common that they are practice-based, fulfil the identified needs of the doctor, and incorporate reflection within the process. These include chart-based audit (facilitated notes review), critical incident analysis, practice-based CME, interactive workshops, PBL and tasked-based learning and critical reading.

A number of Royal Colleges internationally have recognised this and have excellent models for CME which incorporate self-directed and practice-based learning. The Royal College of Physicians and Surgeons of Canada and the Royal Australian Medical College both incorporate note and/or practice review into their CPD.

PROBLEMS WITH LEARNING AND HOW TO OVERCOME THEM

SHIFT WORKING

The 'New Deal' on junior doctors' hours (NHS 1993) and the European Working Time Directive are ensuring that doctors in training are working

Table 1 Learning on shifts: methods of learning which will be more difficult or increasingly common on shift patterns of work

More difficult	Increasingly common
Lectures	Handovers
Departmental meetings	Small group tutorials
Conferences	Case-based teaching
X-ray meetings	Audit
Histology meetings	Role modelling
Journal clubs	Individual learning
	Distance learning

fewer hours than in the past. Campaigners have focused on the risk of long working hours on the health and safety of trainees and their patients. In general, hours have been reduced by changing from traditional on-call rotas to shift patterns of work.

Few researchers have investigated the effect of different work patterns on learning. In general, British research indicates that a closely structured and well-supervised working environment may compensate for a reduction in actual working.[27] A recent Australian review of the literature lends credence to this view, refuting the traditional belief that 'experience' equals learning.[28] More research is needed on ways of achieving changes to the structure and supervision of training which are needed to compensate for shorter periods of duty. Many of the settings and methods traditionally used for teaching and learning will be difficult to deliver in the context of shift working, and other techniques will be increasingly used (Table 1).

PRACTICAL TIPS

GENERAL ADVICE

Learning theory predicts the basic principles of effective learning.

Continuing professional development is more likely to lead to a change in practice when:[3] (i) the learners have diagnosed their own learning needs; (ii) learning is linked to clinical practice; (iii) personal incentive drives the effort to learn; and (iv) learning is re-inforced.

Knowles' adult learning principles can be applied to paediatric medical training (Table 2). Teachers and learners must take motivation into account to: (i) be aware of which factors are motivating us to learn; (ii) ensure that physiological, physical, emotional and social needs are met; and (iii) use positive rather than negative re-inforcement.

However, factors which have been shown to deter uptake of continuing professional development are acknowledged, and must be addressed by trainers and trainees, including: (i) cost (time and money); (ii) dissatisfaction with programmes on offer; (iii) general apathy with respect to education; and (iv) a preference for self-directed learning.

Table 2 The relationship between adult learning theory and medical training

Principle	Example in medical training
Establish an effective learning climate	Trainer is more facilitator than giver of knowledge
Involve learners in mutual planning	Nominate a trainee to be in charge of the teaching programme, in discussion with others
Involve learners in diagnosing their own learning needs	Trainees decide what they need to learn and assign these to each other
Learners encouraged to identify resources	Learners identify learning resources (teachers, books, papers, Internet, patients) to learn about their learning needs
Help learners carry out their learning plans	Expert teachers, library, IT resources provided
Involve learners in evaluating their learning	Learners evaluate their education programme; may assess their learning with feedback

CRITICAL INCIDENT ANALYSIS

Critical incident analysis refers to a framework for recording a critical event which encourages reflection on the events and other people's perspective and identification of learning points to inform future practice.[29] Originally developed for use in adult education, it lends itself very well to medical practice. The terminology, (critical incident), unfortunately carries connotations within the context of the NHS and alternative terminology for the same sort of process includes specific-learning incidents.[30] It is just as useful to apply the framework to events where things went well as it is to use where things did not go exactly as hoped. This allows identification of why they went well so that the skills used can be identified for future similar situations. In practice, however, individuals tend to use the process for events where things went badly (or at least where they perceive them to have gone badly) much more often! The RCPCH allows up to 20 credits per year for reflective note writing and provides a *pro forma* for this. This is much less detailed than the Boud model and does not encourage reflection or consideration of the perspective of others to the same degree. An example of a framework based on Boud can be found in the RCPCH SpR portfolio and Rughani also suggests some frameworks for significant event analyses which readers may find useful.[30]

PORTFOLIOS

Portfolios are being increasingly used to support learning within medical education. Although portfolios are not new, having been widely used in other professions such as architecture and teaching, it is only relatively recently that they have begun to become established in medicine. They have been in use within nursing for a much longer period of time and one of the main features of the UKCC's *Standards for Education and Practice* following registration is the requirement that all practitioners should maintain a portfolio of professional development and continuing education (PREP). Currently, all trainees in paediatrics are expected to maintain a portfolio and there is an RCPCH framework for this. It is likely that revalidation will be largely portfolio-based and consultant appraisal already centres on the development of a folder (portfolio). Since we are all going to be required to develop portfolios, it is important that we use them to their best advantage. At their best, portfolio-based learning should encapsulate the principles of adult learning. It promotes self-directed learning skills and provides a framework for recording learning. This allows for later review of learning in order that it can be implemented in future practice. Portfolios can be entirely self-driven without review by anyone else, but are likely to be more effective when reviewed with someone else – usually an educational supervisor, appraiser or mentor in the context of postgraduate education and CPD.[31] Portfolio learning supported by a co-mentoring group has been used in general practice.[20] In this context, it was felt to encourage active and peer-supported learning as well as meeting learning needs relevant to the individual doctor's practice. With the increasing use of information technology, electronic or Internet-based portfolios are likely to become used more commonly. The Canadian Royal College of Surgeons and Physicians uses an electronic learning log (PCDiary) as part of their maintenance of professional practice (MOCOMP) programme. An Internet-based learning portfolio for residents in obstetrics and gynaecology in Australia was shown to enhance significantly participants' awareness of self-directed learning.[32] Although this was a relatively small study involving only 41 residents over a 4-month period, 7049 patient encounters and 1460 critical incidents of learning were recorded in the study period. This sort of initiative also has the potential to inform training programme planning by facilitating identification of common learning needs for the doctors on the training pro-gramme. In her guide to portfolio-based learning, Challis provides guidance on setting up portfolio learning and some further examples of their use in a medical setting.[31]

COMPUTER-ASSISTED LEARNING

Widespread access to cheap and powerful computers means that computer-assisted learning is accessible to most learners in postgraduate medical education. Computer-assisted learning (CAL) is being increasingly used in undergraduate education and has been shown to be effective in this context.[33] It has been less widely used in postgraduate medical education and CPD, but is likely to become increasingly important especially with the widespread introduction of shift-working making it difficult for trainees to access formal education opportunities. In addition, it is particularly useful for doctors who work in geographically isolated settings. It also offers more potential for self-directed learning than formal didactic teaching, but can have the disadvantage of isolation for the learner. Conversely, Web-based learning groups and E-mail discussion groups potentially allow access to huge numbers of experts around the world allowing participants to learn from their different areas of expertise and differing experiences. Research into the impact of this on patient outcomes and professional practice is needed. A number of interactive patient simulators are available on-line and, although most are American and many adult-based, there are some paediatric ones including a 'virtual' Children's Hospital <http://www.vh.org/VCH> and the opportunity to try and successfully resuscitate on-line <http://www.mdchoice.com/cyberpt/pals/pals.asp>. CD-based learning is also becoming increasingly popular and The Royal College of Obstetrics and Gynaecology have developed a CD-based interactive learning programme for CME. On-line materials should be developed with adult education principles in mind and Zimitat provides some guidance on this.[34]

DISTANCE LEARNING

Distance learning, like CAL, potentially has much to offer doctors working shifts and those who are geographically distant. It may be Web-, CD- or paper-based or contain components of each. Some distance learning courses incorporate regular contact with a tutor and/or other learners while others do not. Distance learning courses which provide tutor and learner contact are thought to be better for learner satisfaction and development.[35] Further work is needed to determine how effective distance learning is at modifying professional practice and health care outcomes.

PROBLEM-BASED AND TASK-BASED LEARNING

Many undergraduate curricula have introduced problem-based learning and there is some evidence to support the view that it is more effective than traditional methods and encourages the development of self-directed learning skills as well as being more enjoyable. Problem-based learning has been less widely used in the postgraduate setting although it may also be effective in this context. A recent review of controlled evaluation studies of problem-based learning in CME did not provide evidence of changes in performance, although there was increased satisfaction with the process compared to other methods.[36] Implementation of a PBL-based CME programme for paediatric asthma management did demonstrate a significant reduction in use and cost of urgent care services in an American health care organisation.[37] General guidance on PBL is provided by Davis.[38] Task-based learning, where tasks undertaken by a doctor are identified and used as a stimulus for learning, has the potential to integrate problem-based learning techniques with clinical practice.[39]

CRITICAL READING OF JOURNALS AND JOURNAL CLUBS

Journal clubs and independent reading have the potential to meet many of the desirable characteristics of adult learning including meeting the individual needs of a given doctor. Teaching of critical appraisal skills should enhance the benefit gained from both journal clubs and individual reading. A recent *Cochrane Review* concluded that there is some evidence teaching critical appraisal skills improves participants' knowledge but that currently there is a paucity of evidence on its effect on decision making or patient care.[40] Currently, RCPCH CPD credits are given for journal clubs, but not for reading journals unless the reading has a specific outcome which is recorded in a reflective note.

Key points for clinical practice

- Effective learning has been shown to improve patient outcomes.

- Traditional didactic education programmes, often based on lectures, have been consistently shown to be less effective than other methods.

- Patient-based learning has been shown to be particularly effective.

- Knowledge of the principles of adult learning helps in understanding why certain types of learning are more effective than others.

- Different individuals learn in different ways – awareness of your own preferred learning style may help you learn more effectively.

- Identifying learning needs is an essential part of planning learning/education.

- Educational supervisors have a key role in facilitating trainees planning learning.

- Portfolios provide a useful framework for structuring learning and have been shown to be an effective means of supporting learning.

- Motivation for learning changes with time and career progression.

- New work patterns make the need to develop self-directed learning skills more important than ever.

- Doctors are more likely to change their practice in response to learning if the desired changes are formally identified and planned.

- Computer-assisted learning and distance learning are likely to be used increasingly in future years because they can be accessed at any time. Further research is needed on their effectiveness.

- Learning is more likely to be effective if we develop the ability to reflect on practice and previous learning.

- A strong evidence base demonstrates that learning must be built into the routine of the normal working day if it is to be effective at improving patient outcomes.

- Time for learning must be recognised in contractual arrangements for all doctors. All doctors must themselves take responsibility for ensuring that they stay up-to-date.

References

1. Madden CA, Mitchell VA. *Professions, Standards and Competence*. Bristol: University of Bristol, 1993.
2. Stanton F, Grant J. Approaches to experiential learning, course delivery and validation in medicine. A background document. *Med Educ* 1999; **33**: 282–297.

3. Grant J, Stanton F. *The Effectiveness of Continuing Professional Development.* Edinburgh: Association for the Study of Medical Education, 2000.
4. McClaren J, Snell L. Type of clinical problem is a determinant of physicians' self-selected learning methods in their practice setting. *J Cont Educ Health Prof* 1998; **18**: 107–118.
5. Ausubel D, Novak J, Hanesian H. *Educational Psychology: A Cognitive View*, 2nd edn. New York: Holt, Rinehart and Winston, 1978.
6. Kolb D. *Experiential Learning: Experience as a Source of Learning and Development.* Englewood Cliffs, NJ: Prentice Hall, 1984.
7. Schon D. *Educating the Reflective Practitioner: Towards a New Design for Teaching and Learning in the Professions.* San Francisco, CA: Jossey-Bass, 1987.
8. Knowles M. *The Adult Learner: A Neglected Species.* Houston, TX: Gulf, 1990.
9. Brookfield S. *Understanding and Facilitating Adult Learning.* Milton Keynes: Open University Press, 1986.
10. Honey P, Mumford A. *Using Your Learning Styles.* Maidenhead: Peter Honey, 1986.
11. Marton F, Saljo R. On qualitative differences in learning II – outcome as a function of the learner's conception of the task. *Br J Educational Psychology* 1976; **46**: 115–127.
12. Newble DI, Entwistle NJ. Learning styles and approaches: implications for medical education. *Med Educ* 1986; **20**: 162–175.
13. Maslow A. *Motivation and Personality.* New York: Harper and Row, 1970.
14. Grant J. Learning needs assessment: assessing the need. *BMJ* 2002; **324**: 156–159.
15. Grant J. Chambers G, Jackson G. (eds) *The Good CPD Guide.* Sutton: Reed Healthcare, 1999.
16. Eve R. Meeting educational needs in general practice: learning with PUNS and DENS. *CME* 1995; **3**: Appendix.
17. Ramsey PG, Wenrich MD, Carline JD, Inui TS, Larson EB, LoGerfo JP. Use of peer ratings to evaluate physician performance. *JAMA* 1993; **269**: 1655–1660.
18. Challis M. AMEE Medical Education Guide No. 19: personal learning plans. *Med Teacher* 2000; **22**: 225–236.
19. Parsell G. Handbooks, learning contracts and senior house officers: a collaborative enterprise. *Postgrad Med J* 1997; **73**: 284–289.
20. Mathers NJ, Challis MC, Howe AC, Field NJ. Portfolios in continuing medical education – effective and efficient? *Med Educ* 1999; **33**: 521–530.
21. Department of Health. *Continuing Professional Development in the New NHS.* London: Department of Health, 1999.
22. Wall D, McAleer S. Teaching the consultant teachers: identifying the core content. *Med Educ* 2000; **34**: 131–138.
23. Davis D, O'Brien MA, Freemantle N, Wolf FM, Mazmanian P, Taylor-Vaisey A. Impact of formal continuing medical education: do conferences, workshops, rounds, and other traditional continuing education activities change physician behavior or health care outcomes? *JAMA* 1999; **282**: 867–874.
24. Abrahamson S, Baron J, Elstein AS *et al.* Continuing medical education for life: eight principles. *Acad Med* 1999; **74**: 1288–1294.
25. O'Brien T, Freemantle N, Oxman AD, Wolf F, Davis DA, Herrin J. Continuing education meetings and workshops: effects on professional practice and health care outcomes (Cochrane Review). *Cochrane Database System Rev* 2001; **2**: CD003030.
26. Mazmanian PE, Johnson RE, Zhang A, Boothby J, Yeatts EJ. Effects of a signature on rates of change: a randomized controlled trial involving continuing education and the commitment-to-change model. *Acad Med* 2001; **76**: 642–646.
27. Anon. *Evaluation of the Reforms to Higher Specialist Training 1996–9.* Milton Keynes: Open University Centre for Medical Education, 2001.
28. Ellis N. *Effects of Work Hours on Learning.* Australian Medical Association, 1998.
29. Boud D, Keogh R, Walker D. (eds) *Reflection. Turning Experience into Learning.* New York: Routledge, 1984.
30. Rughani A. *The GP's Guide to Personal Development Plans.* Oxford: Radcliffe Press, 2000.
31. Challis M. AMEE Medical Education Guide No. 11: Portfolio-based learning and assessment in medical education. *Med Teacher* 1999; **4**: 370–386.
32. Fung MF, Walker M, Fung KF *et al.* An Internet-based learning portfolio in resident education: the KOALA multicentre programme. *Med Educ* 2000; **34**: 474–479.

33. Williams C, Aubin S, Harkin P, Cottrell D. A randomized, controlled, single-blind trial of teaching provided by a computer-based multimedia package versus lecture. *Med Educ* 2001; **35**: 847–854.
34. Zimitat C. Designing effective on-line continuing medical education. *Med Teacher* 2001; **23**: 117–122.
35. Mattheos N, Schittek M, Attstrom R, Lyon HC. Distance learning in academic health education. *Eur J Dent Educ* 2001; **5**: 67–76.
36. Smits PB, Verbeek JH, de Buisonje CD. Problem based learning in continuing medical education: a review of controlled evaluation studies. *BMJ* 2002; **324**: 153–156.
37. Zeitz HJ. Problem based learning: development of a new strategy for effective continuing medical education. *Allergy Asthma Proc* 1999; **20**: 317–321.
38. Davis MH, Harden R. AMEE Medical Education Guide No. 15. Problem based learning: a practical guide. *Med Teacher* 1999; **21**: 130–140.
39. Harden RM, Laidlaw JM, Kerr J, Mitchell H. AMEE Medical Education Booklet No. 7. Task based learning. An educational strategy for undergraduate, postgraduate and continuing medical education. *Med Teacher* 1996; **18**: 7–13.
40. Parkes J, Hyde C, Deeks J, Milne R. Teaching critical appraisal skills in health care settings (Cochrane Review). *Cochrane Database System Rev* 2001; **3**.

T.J. David

14

Paediatric literature review – 2001

To keep this chapter as short as possible, I have decided to provide the name of the first author only. Although the 'convention' would be to give the first three authors, in the context of this chapter the aim is to tell the reader where to find the article. The journal *Archives of Disease in Childhood* has a fetal and neonatal edition as well as a normal one. The pages in the fetal and neonatal edition start with the letter F, *e.g.* F243–F301. The journal *Pediatrics* publishes some electronic articles; the abstract is in the paper journal. These are referenced as in the journal by putting the letter 'e' before the page number, *e.g.* e5.

ALLERGY AND IMMUNOLOGY

Johnston SI *et al.* The protective effect of childhood infections. BMJ 2001; 322: 376–377. *Review. See also pp. 390–395.*

Unsworth DJ. Adrenaline syringes are vastly over prescribed. Arch Dis Child 2001; 84: 410–411. *Review.*

CARDIOVASCULAR

Andrews R *et al.* Outcome of staged reconstructive surgery for hypoplastic left heart syndrome following antenatal diagnosis. Arch Dis Child 2001; 85: 474–477. *Reconstructive surgery has radically altered the prognosis.*

Prof. T.J. David MD PhD FRCP FRCPCH DCH
University Department of Child Health, Booth Hall Children's Hospital, Charlestown Road, Blackley, Manchester M9 7AA, UK
Tel: 0161 220 5536; Fax: 0161 904 9320; E-mail: t.david@netcomuk.co.uk

Mahle WT *et al.* Impact of prenatal diagnosis on survival and early neurologic morbidity in neonates with the hypoplastic left heart syndrome. Pediatrics 2001; 107: 1277–1282. *Prenatal diagnosis has a favourable impact.*

Ringewald JM *et al.* Nonadherence is associated with late rejection in pediatric heart transplant recipients. J Pediatr 2001; 139: 75–78. *Common during adolescence and associated with poor outcome.*

Salmon AP. Hypoplastic left heart syndrome – outcome and management. Arch Dis Child 2001; 85: 450–451. *Review.*

COMMUNITY

Atkinson RL et al. School based programmes on obesity. BMJ 2001; 323: 1018–1019. *Review. See also pp. 1027–1029.*

Bundle A. Health of teenagers in residential care: comparison of data held by care staff with data in community child health records. Arch Dis Child 2001; 84: 10–14. *Important information was not known to the staff.*

Dodd C. Treatment of head lice. BMJ 2001; 323: 1084. *Review.*

Emmons KM et al. A randomised trial to reduce passive smoke exposure in low-income households with young children. Pediatrics 2001; 108: 18–24. *Passive smoking exposure can be reduced.*

Evans JHC. Evidence based management of nocturnal enuresis. BMJ 2001; 323: 1167–1169. *Evidence-based review.*

Jacobson JL et al. Postnatal exposure to PCBs and childhood development. Lancet 2001; 358: 1568–1570. *Review. See also pp. 1602–1607.*

Jewkes F. Prehospital emergency care for children. Arch Dis Child 2001; 84: 103–105. *Review.*

Keen J et al. Drug misusing parents: key points for health professionals. Arch Dis Child 2001; 85: 296–299. *Review.*

Merchant JR et al. Respiratory instability of term and near term healthy newborn infants in car safety seats. Pediatrics 2001; 108: 647–652. *Oxygen saturation declined significantly, with apnoea and bradycardia in some preterm infants.*

Olafsdottir E et al. Randomised controlled trial of infantile colic treated with chiropractic spinal manipulation. Arch Dis Child 2001; 84: 138–124. *Ineffective.*

Puntis JWL. Nutritional support at home and in the community. Arch Dis Child 2001; 84: 295–298. *Review.*

Rudolf MCJ et al. Increasing prevalence of obesity in primary school children: cohort study. BMJ 2001; 322: 1094–1095. *One in five 9-year-olds and one in three 11-year-old girls are overweight.*

Sargent JD et al. Does parental disapproval of smoking prevent adolescents from becoming established smokers? Pediatrics 2001; 108: 1256–1262. *It helps.*

Webb E et al. The health of children in refuges for women victims of domestic violence: cross sectional descriptive survey. BMJ 2001; 323: 210–213. *Specialist health visitors might help.*

ACCIDENTS

American Academy of Paediatrics. Committee on Injury and Poison Prevention. Injuries associated with infant walkers. Pediatrics 2001; 108: 790–792. *Review.*

Barnes PM *et al.* Unnecessary school absence after minor injury: case-control study. BMJ 2001; 323: 1034–1035. *Common.*

Brenner RA *et al.* Where children drown, United States, 1995. Pediatrics 2001; 108: 85–89. *Drowning is the second most common cause of accidental deaths.*

Crouchman M *et al.* A practical outcome scale for paediatric head injury. Arch Dis Child 2001; 84: 120–124. *An expanded adaptation of the Glasgow Outcome Scale.*

Kendrick D *et al.* Randomised controlled trial assessing the impact of increasing information to health visitors about children's injuries. Arch Dis Child 2001; 85: 366–370. *The utility of notifying all injury attendance is questionable.*

Street K *et al.* An unusual cause of injury to an infant. Arch Dis Child 2001; 85: 499. *Face of a baby bitten by a rat.*

Viccellio P *et al.* A prospective multicenter study of cervical spine injury in children. Pediatrics 2001; 108: e20. *Study of 30 cases.*

Warrington SA *et al.* Accidents and resulting injuries in premobile infants: data from the ALSPAC study. Arch Dis Child 2001; 85: 104–107. *Of 1700 falls from beds and settees, there were no head injuries and only one fracture, of a clavicle.*

CHILD ABUSE

Feldman KW et al. The cause of infant and toddler subdural hemorrhage: a prospective study. Pediatrics 2001; 108: 636–645. *Abuse was confirmed in 39 (59%), unintentional injury in 15 (23%), and indeterminate cause in 12 (18%).*

Harrison C et al. Who is failing abused and neglected children? Arch Dis Child 2001; 85: 300–302. *Response to polemic by Speight and Wynne.*

Kairys SW et al. Shaken baby syndrome: rotational cranial injuries – technical report. Pediatrics 2001; 108: 206–210. *Review.*

Labbe J et al. Recent skin injuries in normal children. Pediatrics 2001; 108: 271–276. *The majority of children 9 months and older (76.6%) had at least 1 recent skin injury.*

Rubin DM et al. Pulmonary edema associated with child abuse: case reports and review of the literature. Pediatrics 2001; 108: 769–775. *Report of 2 cases, one after suffocation and one with head injury.*

Shannon P et al. Mechanisms of brain injury in infantile child abuse. Lancet 2001; 358: 686–687. Cervical cord and low brainstem injury, probably due to hyperextension, could lead to apnoea or hypoventilation.

Stanton J et al. Murder misdiagnosed as SIDS: a perpetrator's perspective. Arch Dis Child 2001; 85: 454–459. *Interview material from a woman who murdered 3 children.*

Strathearn L et al. Childhood neglect and cognitive development in extremely low birth weight infants: a prospective study. Pediatrics 2001; 108: 142–151. *Neglect is associated with delayed cognitive development and head growth.*

Trogan I et al. How common is abuse in Greece? Studying cases with femoral fractures. Arch Dis Child 2001; 85: 289–292. *Abuse appears to be unrecognised in Greece.*

Wilson RG. Fabricated or induced illness in children. BMJ 2001; 323: 296–297. *Review.*

HANDICAP

Anonymous. The management of spasticity. Drug Ther Bull 2001; 38: 44–46. *Review.*

Bamiou DE *et al*. Aetiology and clinical presentations of auditory processing disorders – a review. Arch Dis Child 2001; 85: 361–365. *Review.*

Baralle D. Chromosomal aberrations, subtelomeric defects, and mental retardation. Lancet 2001; 358: 7–8. *Review.*

Byard RW. Acute gastric dilation and spastic quadriparesis. J Pediatr 2001; 139: 166. *Fatal case.*

Collet JP *et al*. Hyperbaric oxygen for children with cerebral palsy: a randomised multicentre trial. Arch Dis Child 2001; 85: 160–165. *Did not help.*

Croen LA *et al*. Congenital abnormalities among children with cerebral palsy: more evidence for prenatal antecedents. J Pediatr 2001; 138: 804–810. *Congenital abnormalities were present in 33 (19.2%) children with CP and 21 (4.3%) control children.*

Cunniff C *et al*. Health supervision for children with Down syndrome. Pediatrics 2001; 107: 442–449. *Review.*

Gupta R *et al*. Cerebral palsy: not always what it seems. Arch Dis Child 2001; 85: 356–360. *Review.*

Hoyt CS *et al*. The many challenges of childhood blindness. Arch Dis Child 2001; 85: 452–453. *Review.*

Koman LA *et al*. Botulinum toxin type A neuromuscular blockade in the treatment of equinus foot deformity in cerebral palsy: a multicenter, open-label clinical trial. Pediatrics 2001; 108: 1062–1071. *Safe and effective in focal muscle spasticity.*

Marlow N. A touch of cerebral palsy. Arch Dis Child 2001; 84: F4–F5. *Review.*

Patrick JH *et al*. Therapeutic choices in the locomotor management of the child with cerebral palsy - more luck than judgement? Arch Dis Child 2001; 85: 275–279. *Review*.

Pharoah POD. Cerebral palsy in the surviving twin associated with infant death of the co-twin. Arch Dis Child 2001; 84: F111–F116. *Same sex twin survivors were at higher risk of cerebral palsy*.

Stallard P *et al*. Pain in cognitively impaired, non-communicating children. Arch Dis Child 2001; 85: 460–462. *Everyday pain in children with severe cognitive impairment is common, yet is rarely actively treated*.

IMMUNISATION

Abrahamson JS *et al*. Recommended childhood immunization schedule – United States, January–December 2001. Pediatrics 2001; 107: 202. *Review*.

Ada G. Vaccines and vaccination. N Engl J Med 2001; 345: 1042–1053. *Review*.

Barlow WE *et al*. The risk of seizures after receipt of whole-cell pertussis or measles, mumps, and rubella vaccine. N Engl J Med 2001; 345: 656–661. *Elevated risk of febrile seizures not associated with long-term adverse consequences*.

Choo S *et al*. New pneumococcal vaccines for children. Arch Dis Child 2001; 84: 289–294. *Review*.

Elliman DAC *et al*. MMR vaccine – worries are not justified. Arch Dis Child 2001; 85: 271–274. *Review*.

Elliman D *et al*. MMR vaccine: the continuing saga. BMJ 2001; 322: 183–184. *Review*.

Harnden A *et al*. MMR immunisation. BMJ 2001; 323: 32. *10 minute consultation*.

Kaye JA *et al*. Mumps, measles, and rubella vaccine and the incidence of autism recorded by general practitioners: a time trend analysis. BMJ 2001; 322: 460–463. *No correlation exists between MMR vaccination and autism*.

Maclennan J. Meningococcal group C conjugate vaccines. Arch Dis Child 2001; 84: 383–386. *Review*.

Miller E *et al*. Idiopathic thrombocytopenic purpura and MMR vaccine. Arch Dis Child 2001; 84: 227–229. *Risk within 6 weeks was 1 in 22,300 doses*.

Morrison L. Measles – a minor childhood illness? BMJ 2001; 323: 875. *Report of SSPE*.

Murphy TV *et al*. Intussusception among infants given an oral rotavirus vaccine. N Engl J Med 2001; 344: 564–572. *1 case of intussusception attributable to the vaccine for every 4670 to 9474 infants vaccinated*.

Petrovic M *et al*. Second dose of measles, mumps, and rubella vaccine: questionnaire survey of health professionals. BMJ 2001; 322: 82–85. *Health professionals are poorly informed*.

Skull SA *et al*. Varicella vaccination – a critical review of the evidence. Arch Dis Child 2001; 85: 83–90. *Review*.

INFANT FEEDING

Fewtrell MS *et al*. Randomized trial comparing the efficacy of a novel manual breast pump with a standard electric breast pump in mothers who delivered preterm infants. Pediatrics 2001; 107: 1291–1297. *Manual pump more effective.*

Hamprecht K *et al*. Epidemiology of transmission of cytomegalovirus from mother to preterm infant by breastfeeding. Lancet 2001; 357: 513–518. *Breastfeeding is a source of postnatal infection.*

Hatakka K *et al*. Effect of long term consumption of probiotic milk on infections in children attending day care centres: double blind, randomised trial. BMJ 2001; 322: 1327–1329. *May reduce respiratory infections.*

Jones E *et al*. A randomised controlled trial to compare methods of milk expression after preterm delivery. Arch Dis Child 2001; 85: F91–F95. *Simultaneous pumping is more effective than sequential pumping and breast massage has an additive effect.*

Leeson CPM *et al*. Duration of breast feeding and arterial distensibility in early adult life: population based study. BMJ 2001; 322: 643–647. *The longer the period of breast feeding the less distensible the artery wall in early adult life. See also pp. 625–626.*

Manganaro R *et al*. Incidence of dehydration and hypernatremia in exclusively breast-fed infants. J Pediatr 2001; 139: 673–675. *Of 686 neonates, 53 (7.7%) had a weight loss of greater than or equal to 10% of the birth weight, and 19 also had hypernatraemia.*

Michie CA *et al*. Breast feeding and the risks of viral transmission. Arch Dis Child 2001; 84: 381–382. *Review.*

Oddie S *et al*. Hypernatraemic dehydration and breast feeding: a population study. Arch Dis Child 2001; 85: 318–320. *Unsuccessful breast feeding caused hypernatraemia in 8 of 907 infants re-admitted to hospital in the first month of life.*

Roberts SB. Prevention of hypertension in adulthood by breastfeeding? Lancet 2001; 357: 406–407. *Review. See also pp. 413–419.*

SCREENING AND SURVEILLANCE

Baird G *et al*. Screening and surveillance for autism and pervasive developmental disorders. Arch Dis Child 2001; 84: 468–475. *Review.*

Blair M. The need for and the role of a coordinator in child health surveillance/promotion. Arch Dis Child 2001; 84: 1–5. *Review.*

Fortnum HM. Prevalence of permanent childhood hearing impairment in the United Kingdom and implications for universal neonatal hearing screening: questionnaire based ascertainment study. BMJ 2001; 323: 536–540. *Prevalence of permanent childhood hearing impairment rises over a wider age range than has been reported previously.*

SUDDEN INFANT DEATH SYNDROME (SIDS)

Arnestad M *et al.* Changes in the epidemiological pattern of sudden infant death syndrome in southeast Norway, 1984–1998: implications for future prevention and research. Arch Dis Child 2001; 85: 108–115. *Maternal smoking during pregnancy and maternal age have become more significant risk factors.*

Becroft DMO *et al.* Nasal and intrapulmonary haemorrhage in sudden infant death syndrome. Arch Dis Child 2001; 85: 116–120. *Smothering is a possible factor.*

Horne RSC *et al.* The prone sleeping position impairs arousability in term infants. J Pediatr 2001; 138: 811–816. *May explain why it is a risk factor for SIDS.*

Paris CA *et al.* Risk factors for sudden infant death syndrome: changes associated with sleep position recommendations. J Pediatr 2001; 139: 771–777. *Risk of SIDS increased for low birth weight infants, infants born to mothers who were smokers, unmarried, black, or received limited prenatal care.*

DERMATOLOGY

Davies P et al. Acute nicotine poisoning associated with a traditional remedy for eczema. Arch Dis Child 2001; 85: 500–502. *Dermal absorption of a Bangladeshi remedy.*

Spies M et al. Treatment of extensive toxic epidermal necrolysis in children. Pediatrics 2001; 108: 1162–1168. *Managed successfully in a burn centre.*

ENDOCRINOLOGY

Charmandari E et al. Congenital adrenal hyperplasia: management during critical illness. Arch Dis Child 2001; 85: 26–28. *Best managed with a single intravenous hydrocortisone bolus followed by a constant infusion of hydrocortisone.*

Donaldson M. What is the role of growth-hormone therapy in short children who were small for gestational age? Lancet 2001; 358: 347–348. *Review.*

Eugster E et al. Height outcome in congenital adrenal hyperplasia caused by a 21 hydroxylase deficiency: a meta-analysis. J Pediatr 2001; 138: 26–32. *Adult height is often within 1 SD of target height.*

Menni F et al. Neurologic outcomes of 90 neonates and infants with persistent hyperinsulinemic hypoglycemia. Pediatrics 2001; 107: 476–479. *Important risk to rapidly develop severe mental retardation and epilepsy.*

Munns CFJ et al. Hyperinsulinism and Beckwith-Wiedemann syndrome. Arch Dis Child 2001; 84: F67–F69. *Review.*

DIABETES

Edge JA *et al*. The risk and outcome of cerebral oedema developing during diabetic ketoacidosis. Arch Dis Child 2001; 85: 16–22. *Remains a major problem.*

Hypponen E *et al*. Intake of vitamin D and risk of type 1 diabetes: a birth-cohort study. Lancet 2001; 358: 1500–1503. *Vitamin D supplementation is associated with reduced risk.*

Bennett KE et al. Behaviour and developmental effects of otitis media with effusion into the teens. Arch Dis Child 2001; 85: 91–95. *Deleterious effect on reading ability, verbal IQ, and behaviour problems.*

Butler CC et al. Does early detection of otitis media with effusion prevent delayed language development? Arch Dis Child 2001; 85: 96–103. *Evidence is unclear.*

Chan LS et al. Evidence assessment of management of acute otitis media. II. Research gaps and priorities for future research. Pediatrics 2001; 108: 248–254. *Even the role of antibiotics is unclear. See also pp. 239–247.*

Corbo GM et al. Snoring in 9–15 year old children: risk factors and clinical relevance. Pediatrics 2001; 108: 1149–1154. *Body weight and nasal and pharynx patency seem to be the main determinants of snoring.*

Coyte PC et al. The role of adjuvant adenoidectomy and tonsillectomy in the outcome of the insertion of tympanostomy tubes. N Engl J Med 2001; 344: 1188–1195. *Substantially reduces the likelihood of additional hospitalizations and operations.*

Paradise JL et al. Effect of early or delayed insertion of tympanostomy tubes for persistent otitis media on developmental outcomes at the age of three years. N Engl J Med 2001; 344: 1179–1187. *Prompt insertion does not improve developmental outcomes.*

Roos K et al. Effect of recolonisation with 'interfering' alpha streptococci on recurrences of acute and secretory otitis media in children: randomised placebo controlled trial. BMJ 2001; 322: 210–212. *Good germs may protect against bad ones.*

Armon K *et al*. An evidence and consensus based guideline for acute diarrhoea management. Arch Dis Child 2001; 85: 132–142. *Helpful guidelines.*

Carlsson AK *et al*. Serological screening for celiac disease in healthy 2.5 year old children in Sweden. Pediatrics 2001; 107: 42–45. *Prevalence as high as 1–2%.*

Dignan F. The prognosis of childhood abdominal migraine. Arch Dis Child 2001; 84: 415–418. *Resolved in 61% cases.*

Grant L *et al.* Can pH monitoring reliably detect gastro-oesophageal reflux in preterm infants? Arch Dis Child 2001; 85: F155–F158. *Review.*

Hassall E. Peptic ulcer disease and current approaches to *Helicobacter pylori.* J Pediatr 2001; 138: 462–468. *Review.*

Imrie C *et al.* Is *Helicobacter pylori* infection in childhood a risk factor for gastric cancer? Pediatrics 2001; 107: 373–380. *Review.*

Kline RM *et al.* Enteric-coated, pH-dependent peppermint oil capsules for the treatment of irritable bowel syndrome in children. J Pediatr 2001; 138: 125–128. *76% improved versus 19% on placebo.*

Mitchell DJ *et al.* Simultaneous monitoring of gastric and oesophageal pH reveals limitations of conventional oesophageal pH monitoring in milk fed infants. Arch Dis Child 2001; 84: 273–276. *Buffering by cow's milk may mask reflux detection with pH monitoring.*

Pittock S *et al.* The oral cavity in Crohn's disease. J Pediatr 2001; 138: 767–771. *All children with Crohn's disease should be examined by a dentist.*

Primhak RA *et al.* Alpha-1 antitrypsin deficiency. Arch Dis Child 2001; 85: 2–5. *Review.*

Sharif F *et al.* Liquid paraffin: a reappraisal of its role in the treatment of constipation. Arch Dis Child 2001; 85: 121–124. *Review.*

GENETICS

De Felice C *et al.* Absence of the inferior labial and lingual frenula in Ehlers-Danlos syndrome. Lancet 2001; 357: 1500–1502. *Absence of the inferior labial (100% sensitivity; 99–4% specificity) and lingual frenulum (71.4% sensitivity; 100% specificity) was found to be associated with Ehlers-Danlos syndrome.*

HAEMATOLOGY

Hermansen MC. Nucleated red blood cells in the fetus and newborn. Arch Dis Child 2001; 84: F211–F215. *Review.*

Jacobs BR *et al.* Recombinant tissue plasminogen activator in the treatment of central venous catheter occlusion in children. J Pediatr 2001; 139: 593–596. *Effective in restoring plasminogen activator in the treatment of central venous catheter occlusion in children.*

Kuhne T *et al.* Newly diagnosed idiopathic thrombocytopenic purpura in childhood: an observational study. Lancet 2001; 358: 2122–2125. *2 of 2031 children had intracranial bleeding.*

Saloojee H *et al.* Iron deficiency and impaired child development. BMJ 2001; 323: 1377–1378. *The relation may be causal, but it may not be a priority for intervention. See also pp. 1389–1393.*

Shapiro AD *et al*. Defining the impact of hemophilia: the academic achievement in children with hemophilia study. Pediatrics 2001; 108: e105. *Important association between the number of bleeding episodes and academic achievement.*

van Ommen CH *et al*. Venous thromboembolism in childhood: a prospective two-year registry in The Netherlands. J Pediatr 2001; 139: 676–681. *Almost half of the patients were newborns.*

SICKLE CELL DISEASE

Miller ST *et al*. Silent infarction as a risk factor for overt stroke in children with sickle cell anaemia: a report from the Cooperative Study of Sickle Cell Disease. J Pediatr 2001; 139: 385–390. *Silent infarct is associated with increased stroke risk.*

Wang W *et al*. Neuropsychologic performance in school-aged children with sickle cell disease: a report from the Cooperative Study of Sickle Cell Disease. J Pediatr 2001; 139: 391–397. *Silent infarcts are associated with neuropsychological compromise.*

Wierenga KJJ *et al*. Cerebrovascular complications and parvovirus infection in homozygous sickle cell disease. J Pediatr 2001; 139: 438–442. *Parvovirus causes most aplastic crises in sickle cell disease.*

IMMUNOLOGY

Gaspar HB *et al*. Severe combined immunodeficiency - molecular pathogenesis and diagnosis. Arch Dis Child 2001; 84: 169–173. *Review.*

INFECTIOUS DISEASE

Alan R *et al*. Mannose-binding lectin in prediction of susceptibility to infection. Lancet 2001; 358: 598–600. *Review. See also pp. 614–618.*

Barah F *et al*. Association of human parvovirus B19 infection with acute meningoencephalitis. Lancet 2001; 358: 729–730. *7 of 162 cases of meningoencephalitis had parvovirus.*

Berkley JA *et al*. Diagnosis of acute bacterial meningitis in children at a district hospital in sub-Saharan Africa. Lancet 2001; 357: 1753–1757. *Likely to be missed in a third of cases.*

Booy R *et al*. Reduction in case fatality rate from meningococcal disease associated with improved healthcare delivery. Arch Dis Child 2001; 85: 386–390. *Case fatality fell from 23% in 1992 to 2% in 1997. See also pp. 382–385.*

Breese Hall C. Respiratory syncytial virus and parainfluenza virus. N Engl J Med 2001; 344: 1917–1928. *Review.*

Giebink GS. The prevention of pneumococcal disease in children. N Engl J Med 2001; 345: 1177–1183. *Review.*

Hadzic N. Hepatitis C in pregnancy. Arch Dis Child 2001; 84: F201–F204. *Review.*

Kanegaye JT *et al.* Lumbar puncture in pediatric bacterial meningitis: defining the time interval for recovery of cerebrospinal fluid pathogens after parenteral antibiotic pretreatment. Pediatrics 2001; 108: 1169–1174. *Sterilisation may occur 2–4 h after antibiotics started.*

Nielsen HE *et al.* Diagnostic assessment of haemorrhagic rash and fever. Arch Dis Child 2001; 85: 160–165. *The aetiology was identified in 28%; in 15% it was the meningococcus.*

Rawson H *et al.* Deaths from chickenpox in England and Wales 1995–7: analysis of routine mortality data. BMJ 2001; 323: 1091–1094. *Deaths in adults are increasing.*

Rosenstein NE *et al.* Meningococcal disease. N Engl J Med 2001; 344: 1378–1388. *Review.*

Somekh E *et al.* An intradermal skin test for determination of immunity to varicella. Arch Dis Child 2001; 85: 484–486. *Safe, sensitive, and specific tool.*

Weisse ME. The fourth disease, 1900–2000. Lancet 2001; 357: 299–301. *Review.*

AIDS

Gortmaker SL *et al.* Effect of combination therapy including protease inhibitors on mortality among children and adolescents infected with HIV-1. N Engl J Med 2001; 345: 1522–1528. *Markedly reduced mortality. See also pp. 1568–1569.*

Kline MW *et al.* Adolescents and human immunodeficiency virus infection: the role of the pediatrician in prevention and intervention. Pediatrics 2001; 107: 188–190. *Review.*

MENINGITIS

Bedford H et al. Meningitis in infancy in England and Wales: follow up at age 5 years. BMJ 2001; 323: 533–536. *32 of 1717 (1.8%) died within 5 years and a fifth have a permanent, severe disability.*

Cullington HE. Light eye colour linked to deafness after meningitis. BMJ 2001; 322: 587. *People with light eyes are more prone to deafness after meningitis than those with dark eyes.*

MEDICINE IN THE TROPICS

Betran AP *et al.* Ecological study of effect of breast feeding on infant mortality in Latin America. Lancet 2001; 323: 303–306. *Could substantially reduce infant mortality in Latin America.*

Conroy RM *et al*. Solar disinfection of drinking water protects against cholera in children under 6 years of age. Arch Dis Child 2001; 85: 293–295. *It appears to work.*

Hahn S *et al*. Reduced osmolarity oral rehydration solution for treating dehydration due to diarrhoea in children: systematic review. BMJ 2001; 323: 81–85. *Associated with reduced need for unscheduled intravenous infusions, lower stool volume, and less vomiting. See also pp. 59–60.*

Rahman MM *et al*. Simultaneous zinc and vitamin A supplementation in Bangladeshi children: randomised double blind controlled trial. BMJ 2001; 323: 314–318. *Reduced the prevalence of persistent diarrhoea and dysentery.*

Rosser WW. Paediatric emergency care in developing countries. Lancet 2001; 357: 86–87. *Review.*

MALARIA

Armstrong Schellenberg JRM et al. Effect of large-scale social marketing of insecticide-treated nets on child survival in rural Tanzania. Lancet 2001; 357: 1241–1247. Insecticide-treated nets on child survival in rural Tanzania.

D'Alessandro U. Insecticide treated bed nets to prevent malaria. BMJ 2001; 322: 249–250. The challenge lies in implementation. See also pp. 270–273.

METABOLIC

Chakrapani A *et al*. Detection of inborn errors of metabolism in the newborn. Arch Dis Child 2001; 84: F205–F210. *Review.*

Halberthal M *et al*. Acute hyponatraemia in children admitted to hospital: retrospective analysis of factors contributing to its development and resolution. BMJ 2001; 322: 780–782. *Do not infuse a hypotonic solution if the plasma sodium concentration is less than 138 mmol/l.*

Lund AM *et al*. Feeding difficulties in long-chain 3-hydroxyacyl-CoA dehydrogenase deficiency. Arch Dis Child 2001; 85: 487–488. *Feeding difficulties are common.*

Wraith JE. Ornithine carbamoyltransferase deficiency. Arch Dis Child 2001; 84: 84–88. *Review.*

MISCELLANEOUS

Anttila P et al. Comorbidity of other pains in schoolchildren with migraine or non-migrainous headache. J Pediatr 2001; 138: 176–180. *Children with migraine are more likely to report types of pain other than headaches.*

Bell DS et al. Thirteen year follow-up of children and adolescents with chronic fatigue syndrome. Pediatrics 2001; 107: 994–998. *Twenty percent remain ill with significant symptoms and activity limitation 13 years after illness onset.*

Clark I et al. Salicylates, nitric oxide, malaria, and Reye's syndrome. Lancet 2001; 357: 625–627. *Salicylate may enhance nitric oxide synthase.*

Costello A et al. Reducing global inequalities in child health. Arch Dis Child 2001; 84: 98–102. *Review.*

DiMario FJ. Prospective study of children with cyanotic and pallid breath-holding spells. Pediatrics 2001; 107: 265–269. *Median age of onset 6–12 months, the latest episode tending to occur at 37–42 months.*

Dixon-Woods M et al. Parents' accounts of obtaining a diagnosis of childhood cancer. Lancet 2001; 357: 670–674. *Beware of telling a family categorically that there is nothing wrong with their child.*

Edmunds L et al. Evidence based management of childhood obesity. BMJ 2001; 323: 916–919. *Evidence-based review.*

Faith MS et al. Effects of contingent television on physical activity and television viewing in obese children. Pediatrics 2001; 107: 1043–1048. *The TV only worked if the child pedalled on an exercise bicycle!*

Kemper KJ. Complementary and alternative medicine for children: does it work? Arch Dis Child 2001; 84: 6–9. *Review.*

MacFarlane A et al. Do we need specialist adolescent units in hospitals? BMJ 2001; 322: 941–942. *Review.*

Nelson RM et al. Institutional ethics committees. Pediatrics 2001; 107: 205–209. *Review.*

Pearson HA et al. American pediatrics: milestones at the millennium. Pediatrics 2001; 107: 1482–1491. *Milestones in the history of paediatrics.*

Wade S et al. Infantile colic. BMJ 2001; 323: 437–440. *Evidence-based review.*

NEONATOLOGY

Anderson C. Critical haemoglobin thresholds in premature infants. Arch Dis Child 2001; 84: F146–F148. *Review.*

Andorsky DJ *et al.* Nutritional and other postoperative management of neonates with short bowel syndrome correlates with clinical outcomes. J Pediatr 2001; 139: 27–33. *Early enteral feeding helps. See also pp. 5–7.*

Battin MR *et al.* Neurodevelopmental outcome of infants treated with head cooling and mild hypothermia after perinatal asphyxia. Pediatrics 2001; 107: 480–484. *Supports the safety of hypothermia.*

Baumeister FAM. Glucose monitoring with long-term subcutaneous microdialysis in neonates. Pediatrics 2001; 108: 1187–1192. *Can be used to reduce blood loss of painful stress.*

Benjamin DK *et al.* Bacteremia, central catheters, and neonates: when to pull the line. Pediatrics 2001; 107: 1272–1276. *Once a neonate has 3 positive blood cultures.*

Chiswick M. Parents and end of life decisions in neonatal practice. Arch Dis Child 2001; 85: F1–F3. *Review.*

Clark RH *et al.* Lung injury in neonates: causes, strategies for prevention, and long-term consequences. J Pediatr 2001; 138: 478–486. *Review.*

Davis P *et al.* A randomised controlled trial of two methods of delivering nasal continuous positive airway pressure after extubation to infants weighing less than 1000 g: binasal (Hudson) versus single nasal prongs. Arch Dis Child 2001; 85: F82–F85. *Binasal prongs are more effective in preventing failure of extubation.*

Davis PJ *et al.* Meconium aspiration syndrome and extracorporeal membrane oxygenation. Arch Dis Child 2001; 84: F1–F3. *Review.*

Dennery PA *et al.* Neonatal hyperbilirubinemia. N Engl J Med 2001; 344: 581–590. *Review.*

Embleton ND *et al.* Foot length, an accurate predictor of nasotracheal tube length in neonates. Arch Dis Child 2001; 85: F60–F64. *A reliable and reproducible predictor.*

Kaufman D *et al.* Fluconazole prophylaxis against fungal colonization and infection in preterm infants. N Engl J Med 2001; 345: 1660–1666. *Effective in preventing fungal colonization and invasive fungal infection.*

Kennedy CR *et al.* Randomized, controlled trial of acetazolamide and furosemide in posthemorrhagic ventricular dilation in infancy: follow-up at 1 year. Pediatrics 2001; 108: 597–607. *Ineffective in decreasing the rate of shunt placement and associated with increased neurological morbidity.*

Kimberlin DW *et al.* Safety and efficacy of high-dose intravenous acyclovir in the management of neonatal herpes simplex virus infections. Pediatrics 2001; 108: 230–238. *Appears reasonably safe and effective. For natural history of neonatal herpes see pp. 223–229.*

Kumar D *et al.* Vitamin K status of premature infants: implications for current recommendations. Pediatrics 2001; 108: 1117–1122. *Vitamin K levels in premature infants directly reflect vitamin K intakes.*

Lee TWR *et al.* Routine neonatal examination: effectiveness of trainee paediatrician compared with advanced neonatal nurse practitioner. Arch Dis Child 2001; 85: F100–F104. *Nurses are more effective. This also applies to resuscitation, see pp. F96–F99.*

Maalouf EF *et al.* Comparison of findings on cranial ultrasound and magnetic resonance imaging in preterm infants. Pediatrics 2001; 107: 719–727. *Each method has its own advantages/disadvantages.*

Maisels MJ *et al.* Neonatal jaundice and kernicterus. Pediatrics 2001; 108: 763–765. *Review.*

McIntosh N *et al.* High or low oxygen saturation for the preterm baby. Arch Dis Child 2001; 84: F149–F150. *Comments by 2 neonatologists.*

Moster D *et al.* The association of Apgar score with subsequent death and cerebral palsy: a population-based study in term infants. J Pediatr 2001; 138: 798–803. *Scores of 0–3 were associated with a 386-fold increased risk of neonatal death.*

Murphy BP *et al*. Impaired cerebral cortical gray matter growth after treatment with dexamethasone for neonatal chronic lung disease. Pediatrics 2001; 107: 217–226. *Impairment in brain growth secondary to dexamethasone therapy.*

Nadroo AM *et al*. Death as a complication of peripherally inserted central catheters in neonates. J Pediatr 2001; 138: 599–601. *Uniform guidelines are needed.*

Narendra A *et al*. Nephrocalcinosis in preterm babies. Arch Dis Child 2001; 85: F207–F213. *16% of babies born at less than 32 weeks developed nephrocalcinosis.*

Ng PC *et al*. Randomised controlled study of oral erythromycin for treatment of gastrointestinal dysmotility in preterm infants. Arch Dis Child 2001; 84: F177–F182. *Effective but safety not yet established.*

Pal BR *et al*. Frontal horn thin walled cysts in preterm neonates are benign. Arch Dis Child 2001; 85: F187–F193. *10 of 11 survivors had a normal outcome.*

Papile LA. The Apgar score in the 21st century. N Engl J Med 2001; 344: 519–520. *Review. See also pp. 467–471.*

Pearson DL *et al*. Neonatal pulmonary hypertension. Urea-cycle intermediates, nitric oxide production, and carbamoyl-phosphate synthetase function. N Engl J Med 2001; 344: 1832–1838. *Inadequate production of nitric oxide is involved in the pathogenesis.*

Perlman JM. Neurobehavioral deficits in premature graduates of intensive care – potential medical and neonatal environmental risk factors. Pediatrics 2001; 108: 1339–1348. *Review.*

Rutter N. Can we use methadone for analgesia in neonates? Arch Dis Child 2001; 85: F79–F81. *Review.*

Saarenmaa E *et al*. Ketamine for procedural pain relief in newborn infants. Arch Dis Child 2001; 85: F53–F56. *Ineffective in the doses used.*

Saugstad OD. Is oxygen more toxic than currently believed? Pediatrics 2001; 108: 1203–1205. *Review.*

Schmidt B *et al*. Long-term effects of indomethacin prophylaxis in extremely low birth weight infants. N Engl J Med 2001; 344: 1966–1972. *Does not improve survival without neurosensory impairment.*

Sohn AH *et al*. Prevalence of nosocomial infections in neonatal intensive care unit patients: results from the first national point-prevalence survey. J Pediatr 2001; 139: 821–827. *Documents the high prevalence.*

Valaes T. Problems with prediction of neonatal hyperbilirubinemia. Pediatrics 2001; 108: 175–177. *Review. See also pp. 31–39.*

NEPHROLOGY

Cascio S *et al*. Bacterial colonization of the prepuce in boys with vesicoureteral reflux who receive antibiotic prophylaxis. J Pediatr 2001; 139: 160–162. *The preputial sac is an important reservoir for uropathic organisms.*

deBuys Roessingh AS *et al*. Dipstick measurements of urine specific gravity are unreliable. Arch Dis Child 2001; 85: 155–157. *Only refractometry gives reliable results.*

Deshpande PV *et al*. An audit of RCP guidelines on DMSA scanning after urinary tract infection. Arch Dis Child 2001; 84: 324–327. *DMSA scans can be omitted in children over 1 year with first simple UTI not sufficiently ill to be admitted to hospital.*

Elliott EJ *et al*. Nationwide study of haemolytic uraemic syndrome: clinical, microbiological, and epidemiological features. Arch Dis Child 2001; 85: 125–131. *Study of 98 cases.*

Eriksson KJ *et al*. Acute neurology and neurophysiology of haemolytic-uraemic syndrome. Arch Dis Child 2001; 84: 434–345. *CNS affected in 30% of cases.*

Hulton SA. Evaluation of urinary tract calculi in children. Arch Dis Child 2001; 84: 320–323. *Review.*

Smellie JM *et al*. Medical versus surgical treatment in children with severe bilateral vesicouretic reflux and bilateral nephropathy: a randomised trial. Lancet 2001; 357: 1329–1333. *Outcome similar in both groups. See also pp. 1309–1310.*

Tran D *et al*. Short-course versus conventional length antimicrobial therapy for uncomplicated lower urinary tract infections in children: a meta-analysis of 1279 patients. J Pediatr 2001; 139: 93–99. *Single-dose amoxicillin is inadequate.*

NEUROLOGY

Biggar WD et al. Deflazacort treatment of Duchenne muscular dystrophy. J Pediatr 2001; 138: 45–50. *May preserve gross motor and pulmonary function but 10/30 had cataracts.*

Bitsori M et al. Facial nerve palsy associated with *Rickettsia conorii* infection. Arch Dis Child 2001; 85: 54–55. *Report of 2 cases.*

Chumas P et al. Hydrocephalus – what's new? Arch Dis Child 2001; 85: F149–F154. *Review.*

Essex C et al. Late diagnosis of Duchenne's muscular dystrophy presenting as global developmental delay. BMJ 2001; 323: 37–38. *Report of 3 cases.*

Glasgow JFT et al. Reye syndrome – insights on causation and prognosis. Arch Dis Child 2001; 85: 351–353. *Review.*

Kirkham FJ. Non-traumatic coma in children. Arch Dis Child 2001; 85: 303–312. *Review.*

Riordan M. Investigation and treatment of facial paralysis. Arch Dis Child 2001; 84: 286–287. *Review.*

Tang T et al. A painful hip as a presentation of Guillain-Barré syndrome in children. BMJ 2001; 322: 149–150. *Case report.*

Zuberi SM et al. Ion channels and neurology. Arch Dis Child 2001; 84: 277–280. *Review.*

EPILEPSY

Anonymous. Managing childhood epilepsy. Drug Ther Bull 2001; 39: 12–16. *Review.*

Austin JK *et al.* Behaviour problems in children before first recognized seizures. Pediatrics 2001; 107: 115–122. *Suggests the two may be part of a single disorder.*

Besag FMC. Tonic seizures are a particular risk factor for drowning in people with epilepsy. BMJ 2001; 322: 975–976. *Report on a 14-year-old. See also pp. 940–941.*

Callenbach PMC *et al.* Mortality risk in children with epilepsy: the Dutch study of epilepsy in childhood. Pediatrics 2001; 107: 1259–1263. *Children who have symptomatic epilepsy have a 20-fold increased mortality risk.*

Koul R *et al.* Vigabatrin associated retinal dysfunction in children with epilepsy. Arch Dis Child 2001; 85: 469–473. *Vigabatrin can cause eye damage.*

Nordli DR *et al.* Experience with the ketogenic diet in infants. Pediatrics 2001; 108: 129–133. *Safe and effective treatment.*

Offringa M *et al.* Evidence based management of seizures associated with fever. BMJ 2001; 323: 1111–1114. *Evidence-based review.*

Post JC *et al.* Panaylotopoulos syndrome: a common and benign childhood epilepsy. Lancet 2001; 357: 821–824. *Review.*

NUTRITION

Carvalho NF et al. Severe nutritional deficiencies in toddlers resulting from health food milk alternatives. Pediatrics 2001; 107: e46. *Report of 2 cases and literature review.*

Tomashek KM et al. Nutritional rickets in Georgia. Pediatrics 2001; 107: e45. *Review.*

Wells JCK. A critique of the expression of paediatric body composition data. Arch Dis Child 2001; 85: 67–72. *Review.*

ORTHOPAEDICS

Boutis K et al. Sensitivity of a clinical examination to predict need for radiography in children with ankle injuries: a prospective study. Lancet 2001; 358: 2118–2121. *Skilled clinical examination identifies high risk diagnoses.*

Kendall JM. Multicentre randomised controlled trial of nasal diamorphine for analgesia in children and teenagers with clinical fractures. BMJ 2001; 322: 261–265. *The preferred method of pain relief.*

Margetts BM et al. The incidence and distribution of Legg-Calve-Perthes' disease in Liverpool, 1982–95. Arch Dis Child 2001; 84: 351–354. *Association with deprivation.*

Specker BL. The significance of high bone density in children. J Pediatr 2001; 139: 473–475. *Review. See also pp. 494–526.*

PSYCHIATRY

Accardo P *et al.* What's all the fuss about Ritalin? J Pediatr 2001; 138: 6–9. *Review.*

Bolton PF *et al.* Association between idiopathic infantile macrocephaly and autism spectrum disorders. Lancet 2001; 358: 726–727. *Macrocephaly was associated with an increased risk of developing autism.*

Coniglio SJ *et al.* A randomized, double-blind, placebo-controlled trial of single-dose intravenous secretin as treatment for children with autism. J Pediatr 2001; 138: 649–655. *No significant effect.*

Fombonne E. Is there an epidemic of autism? Pediatrics 2001; 107: 411–413. *Review.*

Guevara JP *et al.* Evidence based management of attention deficit hyperactivity disorder. BMJ 2001; 323: 1232–1235. *Evidence-based review.*

Hill P *et al.* An auditable protocol for treating attention deficit/hyperactivity disorder. Arch Dis Child 2001; 84: 404–409. *Derived from standard recommendations.*

Walkup JT *et al.* Fluvoxamine for the treatment of anxiety disorders in children and adolescents. N Engl J Med 2001; 344: 1279–1285. *Effective treatment.*

RESPIRATORY

Castro-Rodriguez JA et al. Relation of two different subtypes of croup before age three to wheezing, atopy, and pulmonary function during childhood: a prospective study. Pediatrics 2001; 170: 512–518. *A subset is at increased risk of subsequent recurrent lower respiratory tract obstruction.*

Russell G. Community acquired pneumonia. Arch Dis Child 2001; 85: 445–446. *Review.*

ASTHMA

Cane RS *et al.* Parents' interpretations of children's respiratory symptoms on video. Arch Dis Child 2001; 84: 31–34. *The correct labelling of wheeze was only 59%.*

Chavasse RJ *et al*. Persistent wheezing in infants with an atopic tendency responds to inhaled fluticasone. Arch Dis Child 2001; 85: 143–148. *Small sample size, short-trial, potential side effects uncertain.*

Kuehni CE *et al*. Are all wheezing disorders in very young (preschool) children increasing in prevalence? Lancet 2001; 357: 1821–1825. *Doubling in the prevalence in the last 8 years.*

Lanphear BP *et al*. Residential exposures associated with asthma in US children. Pediatrics 2001; 107: 505–511. *In theory, 39% of asthma could be prevented by avoiding exposures to indoor pollutants and allergens.*

McPherson A *et al*. Double click for health: the role of multimedia in asthma education. Arch Dis Child 2001; 85: 447–449. *Review.*

Patel L *et al*. Symptomatic adrenal insufficiency during inhaled corticosteroid treatment. Arch Dis Child 2001; 85: 330–334. *Report of 8 cases, all associated with standard recommended dosages.*

Qureshi F *et al*. Comparative efficacy of oral dexamethasone versus oral prednisone in acute pediatric asthma. J Pediatr 2001; 139: 20–26. *2 doses of dexamethasone provide similar efficacy with improved compliance and fewer side effects than 5 doses of prednisone.*

Roland DIM *et al*. Oxygen treatment for acute severe asthma. BMJ 2001; 323: 98–100. *Oxygen treatment for acute severe asthma.*

CYSTIC FIBROSIS

Chen JS *et al*. Endemicity and inter-city spread of *Burkholderia cepacia* genomovar III in cystic fibrosis. J Pediatr 2001; 139: 643–649. Burkholderia *may remain endemic in cystic fibrosis centres for many years.*

Coates AL. What is the cystic fibrosis clinician supposed to do with human recombinant dornase alfa? J Pediatr 2001; 139: 768–770. *Uncertainty remains. See pp. 813–820.*

Cunningham S *et al*. Bronchoconstriction following nebulised colistin in cystic fibrosis. Arch Dis Child 2001; 84: 432–443. *Occurred in 20 of 58 children.*

Doull IJM. Recent advances in cystic fibrosis. Arch Dis Child 2001; 85: 62–66. *Review.*

Equi AC *et al*. Use of cough swabs in a cystic fibrosis clinic. Arch Dis Child 2001; 85: 438–439. *A positive cough swab is a strong predictor of sputum culture. A negative cough swab does not rule out infection.*

Farrell PM *et al*. Early diagnosis of cystic fibrosis through neonatal screening prevents severe malnutrition and improves long-term growth. Paediatrics 2001; 107: 1–13. *Severe malnutrition persists after delayed diagnosis and catch-up may not be possible.*

Hamilton JW. Gentamicin in pharmacogenetic approach to treatment of cystic fibrosis. Lancet 2001; 358: 2014–2016. *Review.*

Hardin DS *et al*. Normal bone mineral density in cystic fibrosis. Arch Dis Child 2001; 84: 363–368. *Osteopenia and osteoporosis may be caused more by malnutrition and chronic use of intravenous or oral corticosteroids than by a CF-related inherent defect.*

Jones AM *et al*. Spread of a multiresistant strain of *Pseudomonas aeruginosa* in an adult cystic fibrosis clinic. Lancet 2001; 358: 557–560. *Cross infection a major problem. See also pp. 522–523.*

Merelle ME *et al*. Cystic fibrosis presenting with intracerebral haemorrhage. Lancet 2001; 358: 1960. *Due to vitamin K deficiency.*

Miall LS *et al*. Methicillin resistant *Staphylococcus aureus* (MRSA) infection in cystic fibrosis. Arch Dis Child 2001; 84: 160–162. *Associated with more severe disease.*

Nixon GM *et al*. Clinical outcome after *Pseudomonas aeruginosa* infection in cystic fibrosis. J Pediatr 2001; 138: 699–704. *Acquisition of* P. aeruginosa *was associated with increased morbidity and mortality.*

Ranganathan SC *et al*. Airway function in infants newly diagnosed with cystic fibrosis. Lancet 2001; 358: 1964–1965. *Abnormalities were identified even in those with no respiratory symptoms.*

Wang SS *et al*. Early diagnosis of cystic fibrosis in the newborn period and risk of *Pseudomonas aeruginosa* acquisition in the first 10 years of life: a registry-based longitudinal study. Pediatrics 2001; 107: 274–280. *Early asymptomatic diagnosis of CF did not affect* P. aeruginosa *acquisition.*

RHEUMATOLOGY

Malleson PN *et al*. Chronic musculoskeletal and other idiopathic pain syndromes. Arch Dis Child 2001; 84: 189–192. *Review.*

Mukamel M *et al*. New insight into calcinosis of juvenile dermatomyositis: a study of composition and treatment. J Pediatr 2001; 138: 763–766. *Alendronate can be an effective treatment.*

SURGERY

DeFelice C *et al*. Infantile hypertrophic pyloric stenosis and asymptomatic joint hypermobility. J Pediatr 2001; 138: 596–598. *A significant association is claimed.*

Hedback G *et al*. The epidemiology of infantile hypertrophic pyloric stenosis in Sweden 1987–96. Arch Dis Child 2001; 85: 379–381. *The declining incidence and geographical difference suggest that environmental factors are of importance in this disorder.*

Kenny SE *et al*. Double blind randomised controlled trial of topical glyceryl trinitrate in anal fissure. Arch Dis Child 2001; 85: 404–407. *The drug is ineffective but a nurse-based treatment programme worked.*

Mahon BE *et al*. Maternal and infant use of erythromycin and other macrolide antibiotics as risk factors for infantile hypertrophic pyloric stenosis. J Pediatr 2001; 139: 380–384. *Confirms association.*

Preece JM *et al*. Acute urinary retention: an unusual presentation of acute appendicitis in a 3 year old boy. Arch Dis Child 2001; 84: 269. *Single case.*

TROPICAL MEDICINE see MEDICINE IN THE TROPICS

Index

The Recent Advances Series

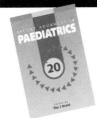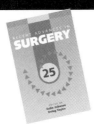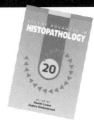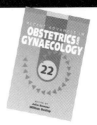

Other Titles in the Recent Advances Series

> You can set up a *standing order* and receive the next edition as soon as it is published.
> Just call +44 (0)1235 465 500

Recent Advances in Surgery 25
Edited by Colin Johnson & Irving Taylor
£32.95, 1-85315-508-X, pbk, 250pp, May 2002 **www.rsm.ac.uk/pub/bkjohnson.htm**

Recent Advances in Histopathology 20
Edited by James Underwood & David Lowe
£32.95, 1-85315-511-X, pbk, 250pp, May 2003 **www.rsm.ac.uk/pub/bkunderwood.htm**

Recent Advances in Obstetrics and Gynaecology 22
Edited by John Bonnar & William Dunlop
£35.00, 1-85315-529-2, pbk, 250pp, February 2003 **www.rsm.ac.uk/pub/bkbonner.htm**

Other books available from RSM Press

Our publications span a range of topics - in particular we publish many titles in the areas of healthcare management and primary care, and also a number of well-received postgraduate exam texts.

Paediatric Radiology for MRCPCH and FRCR, *C Schelvan, A Copeman, J Young, J Davis*
'This book is clearly written and contains a lot of information.' *Pediatric Radiology*
'This book is very clearly set out with a useful initial section of interpretation, rules and tools with each of the 100 or so cases. The book will be a useful aid to doctors training in their examinations, and, indeed, could be a useful text for CPD consultants.' *Postgraduate Medical Journal*
£17.50, 256pp, 1-85315-466-0, pbk, January 2002
Read sample questions FREE online at www.rsm.ac.uk/pub/bkschelvan.htm

100 Grey Cases for the MRCPCH, *N Barakat*
These cases have been written by an experienced paediatrician familiar with the format of the examination, and test clinical and decision-making skills.
£15.95, 200pp, 1-85315-524-1, pbk, February 2003 **www.rsm.ac.uk/pub/bkbaraka3.htm**

Law for Doctors, Principles and practicalities, 2nd Edition, *M Branthwaite & N Beresford*
Praise for the first edition
'An excellent introduction ... this book stands out from the rest.' *Medical Litigation*
'This is an excellent book. Every doctor would benefit from reading it.' *British Journal of Anaesthesia*
£9.50, 96pp, 1-85315-540-3, pbk, January 2003
Read a sample chapter FREE online at www.rsm.ac.uk/pub/bkbranth.htm

Medical Evidence, A handbook for doctors, edited by *RV Clements* et al
'This book is a marvellous repository of information and good advice for any doctors preparing themselves for a court appearance, for whatever reason.' *Health Service Journal*
£18.50, 130pp, 1-85315-387-7, pbk, April 2001 www.rsm.ac.uk/pub/bkclements.htm

How to order

Contact our distributors
Marston Book Services
PO Box 269, Abingdon
Oxfordshire, OX14 4YN
Tel +44 (0)1235 465 500
Fax +44 (0)1235 465 555

online at
www.rsmpress.co.uk

From our catalogue
To receive a catalogue featuring all our books and journals please e-mail
rsmpublishing@rsm.ac.uk or
call +44 (0)20 7290 3926